MANUAL OF
HEALTHY
LONGEVITY
& WELLBEING

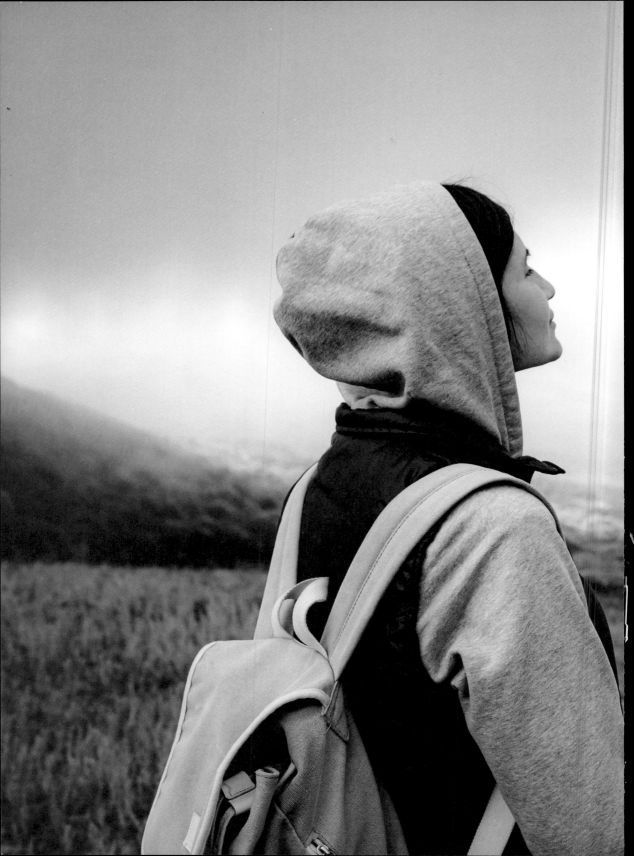

MANUAL OF
HEALTHY LONGEVITY & WELLBEING

A THREE STEP PLAN

PROFESSOR LUIGI FONTANA

MD, PHD, FRACP
Scientific Director,
Charles Perkins Centre Royal Prince Alfred Clinic
Director,
Healthy Longevity Research and Clinical Program
University of Sydney

Hardie Grant

BOOKS

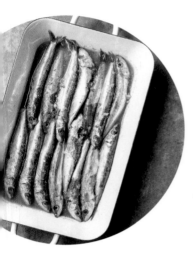

CONTENTS

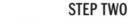

INTRODUCTION VI

STEP ONE
NUTRITION FOR LONGEVITY 1
BEYOND WEIGHT LOSS 3
THE MODERN LONGEVITY DIET 9
RECIPES 21

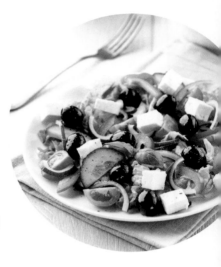

STEP TWO
EXERCISE: A POWERFUL MEDICINE 133
THE IMPORTANCE OF EXERCISE 135
AEROBIC EXERCISE 140
FITNESS 146
STRENGTH TRAINING 158
ALL IN BALANCE 182
EAST MEETS WEST 188
TAKE A BREATH 196

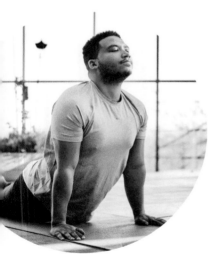

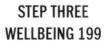

STEP THREE
WELLBEING 199
ALL ABOUT REST 203
MINDFULNESS 205
ONE STEP AT A TIME 212

ACKNOWLEDGEMENTS 214
ABOUT THE AUTHOR 215

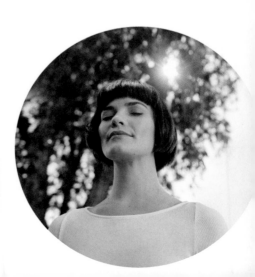

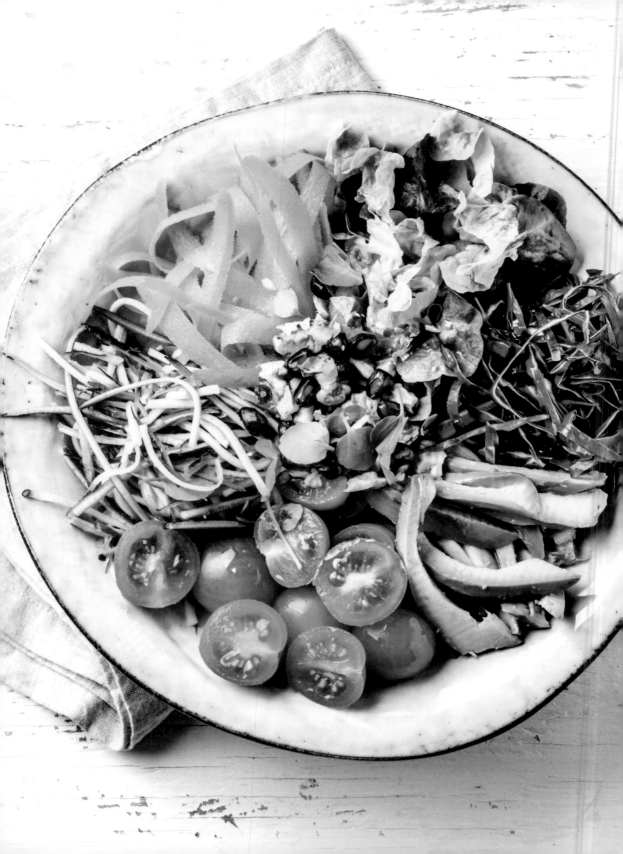

INTRODUCTION

The aim of this new book is to provide a practical guide to the science and philosophy of healthy longevity and wellbeing.

A companion book *The Path to Longevity* containing in-depth theoretical knowledge was published in 2020. That book was a comprehensive description of the interventions and mechanisms promoting physical, mental, emotional and spiritual wellbeing. It was designed to explain, review, and explore both old and present knowledge and included many recent scientific developments and advances in the science of health promotion, disease prevention and healthy longevity.

This *Manual of Healthy Longevity & Wellbeing* has been compiled, along with illustrations throughout, to provide the reader with the practical tools to implement the concepts outlined in my earlier book. My patients, students and followers often express their desire to understand what they should eat, how they should use ingredients to create healthy and tasty recipes, and what type of exercises and meditative techniques they should implement to boost their physical, mental, emotional and spiritual health. I hope that this book will help satisfy their requests. And for those who find my books and scientific articles too difficult and complex, this practical *Manual of Healthy Longevity & Wellbeing* shares the simple and holistic steps we can take for healthy longevity.

STEP ONE

NUTRITION FOR LONGEVITY

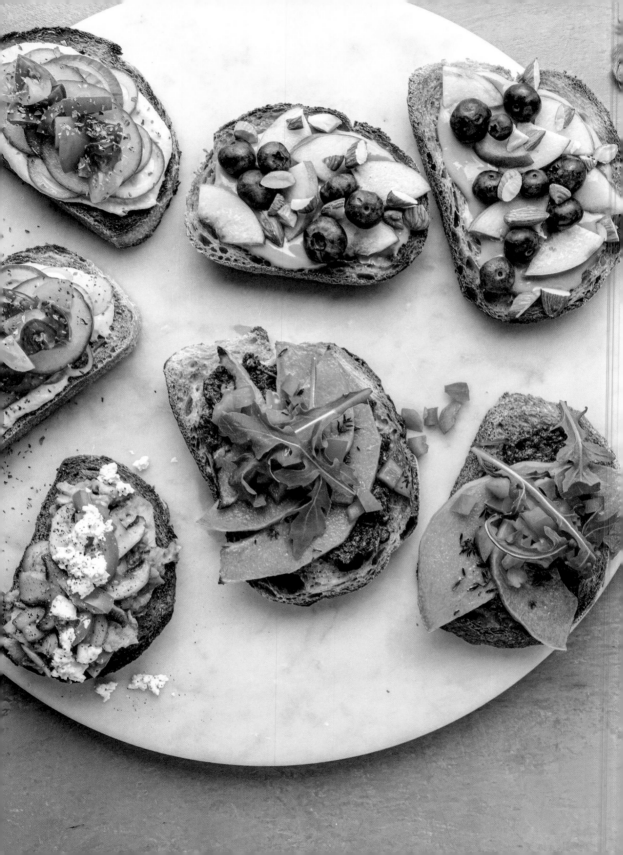

BEYOND WEIGHT LOSS

There are lots of different ideas when it comes to good nutrition, and you've probably heard about most of them: keto, paleo, low carb, high protein, the Zone, Dukan, 5:2, 16:8 … New variations of these ideas seem to come into favour each month, and any number of celebrity endorsements pushes them into the spotlight.

You'll always find people who say these eating plans work for them, and probably none of them will be lying to you. If your sole purpose is to lose weight, I could offer you a number of eating plans that would achieve excellent results. What they won't do, however, is make a long-term investment in the essential nutrition, and other lifestyle interventions, that will both *maximise your health* and *prolong your life*.

The plan outlined in the following pages is backed by years of scientific research, clinical trials and practice. Many ideas are ones with which you might already be familiar, but here they're integrated in a way that has been scientifically proven to help prevent chronic disease and maximise health. These are some of the biggest steps you can take to improve your long-term wellbeing.

START WITH THE SCIENCE

It should not come as news that being overweight puts you at a higher risk of getting sick and ageing faster. Consuming more food, and therefore calories, than we need to move and think, and for our bodies to perform basic functions, means those excess calories are dumped into fat cells.

Those enlarged fat cells then produce inflammation and hormones that increase the risk of developing many serious and debilitating chronic illnesses. I'm talking about type 2 diabetes, cancer, dementia, and heart, liver and kidney disease, but there are more.

CHECK YOUR BODY WEIGHT

BMI AND WHAT'S A NORMAL BMI?

BMI is a good start to assessing your health status. BMI (body mass index) is a simple measure of body fat. People within a normal weight limit have a BMI of between 18.5 and 25. Anything over 25 is overweight; over 30 and you're considered obese. Below 18.5 is underweight.

Of course, maintaining a healthy BMI of between 18.5 and 25 doesn't necessarily mean you'll live a long and healthy life. Slim people are not necessarily fit, while someone who is larger may, in fact, have a predominance of muscle with very little abdominal fat.

It's essential to combine a healthy BMI with a healthy diet and regular exercise to prevent chronic illness and live a longer life.

WORK OUT YOUR OWN BMI

Divide your weight in kilograms by your height in metres. Then divide the answer by your height again. So, if you're 70 kg and 1.75 m tall, divide 70 by 1.75. The answer is 40, which you divide by 1.75 again to get 22.9. That figure is your BMI. In this case, at 22.9, it's in the healthy range. If you are using pounds and inches, either use a metric converter or apply this formula to convert to metric: weight (pounds) × 0.45 / height (inches) × 0.025.

WHY YOU SHOULD MONITOR YOUR WEIGHT

Even if you have a normal BMI, it's important to monitor weight fluctuations. For every kilogram (2 pounds) of weight gained after your eighteenth birthday, the odds of living a long and healthy life are thought to decrease by 5 per cent.

Even small weight gains can compound and take someone from healthy to overweight, when it becomes much harder to lose. Dealing with weight gains quickly stops them from spiralling to a point that is much harder to reset to normal.

If you don't reset your diet it is likely you will suffer from the slow creep of weight gain, where it is incredibly easy to gain a kilogram or couple of pounds every year.

WAIST MEASURES

Ideally Australian, European and North American men should have a waist measurement of less than 94 cm (37 inches); for women it should be less than 80 cm (31½ inches). For South Asian and Chinese men that measurement is less than 90 cm (35½ inches) and for women it's 80 cm (31½ inches). Remember that unlike for body weight, the lower your waist measurement the better.

WATCH YOUR WAIST

BMI isn't the only measure of body fat. In fact, where body fat is located is an excellent predictor of health. The worst type is belly fat, which accumulates when people eat too much and lead a sedentary lifestyle. (It used to be that this was a problem mainly for men – women tended to gain weight around the hips. This, however, is changing, just look around you.)

If you've had to increase the size of your pants or skirts since your late teens, you have increased abdominal fat. In an ideal world, your abdomen would be flat with its muscles showing. There should be no extra fat that can be pinched.

But don't despair, because every time you lose a little off your waist measurement, you are making a real and significant reduction in harmful belly fat.

Even a modest weight loss of between 8 and 10 per cent can mean losing about 40 per cent of visceral fat, like belly fat, which can have a major improvement in the way your heart and lungs function. It has also been shown to reduce the risk of type 2 diabetes, hypertension, heart disease and cancer.

LOSING WEIGHT

For most people, losing 10 per cent of their body weight isn't that much. Aim for slow and steady progress: try to reach your 10 per cent target in six to 12 months. Once you've maintained your new weight for six months, make yourself another weight-loss goal if you still need to lose more.

But just dieting or eating fewer calories or fasting on a 5:2 regime does not guarantee that you will lose weight. Exercise is an important part of the equation.

It is, of course, possible to lose weight faster than this. But very low calorie diets can sometimes cause serious nutritional inadequacies. At their worst, they can even cause malnutrition. There's also a much higher possibility of regaining the weight at some stage.

KEEPING IT OFF

If you've ever lost weight before, you probably know that the real challenge is maintaining your new thinner self. Regaining the kilos is usually due to a slowing of metabolism, but studies have shown that adding endurance and strength training (*see* Step Two: Exercise) to your weight-loss routine cancels this out.

IT'S NOT ONLY ABOUT WEIGHT

As a society, we have become obsessed by losing weight. It's seen as the end goal. But the concept of successful ageing and healthy longevity goes well beyond weight loss. Your diet has to provide full nutrition and be part of an integrated healthy lifestyle that includes regular exercise, good sleep, meditation and some breathing techniques. Whenever you're assessing how you can make investments in your health, it should go well beyond just dropping extra kilos. You need to do all you can to avoid developing chronic illness as you age, so as to live a longer, healthier and fulfilling life.

FASTING AND OTHER 'TRICKS'

WHAT IS HEALTHY FASTING?

Lots of people have recently tried the 5:2 diet. The idea is that you reduce calories drastically for two days each week, then, on the other five days, eat normally. That can be an effective way to reduce the calories you consume overall and your body weight.

Unfortunately many think that the 'eat what you like' philosophy applies to the five days of eating normally which inevitably leads to people consuming junk food that offers no nutritional value and can have detrimental effects on your metabolic and gut health and increase the risk of developing chronic illnesses. Alternatively they eat large meals and snack in between meals on their non-fasting days, negating the point of the fasting days.

There are potential benefits to fasting, you just need to do it properly by making a healthy diet your new normal.

The 16:8 diet (time-restricted eating) may work better for some people. It involves restricting daily food intake to the hours between 7 am and 2 pm (i.e. eight hours of the day). This does back up some old ways of thinking, particularly when it comes to breakfast being the most important meal of the day.

This way of eating involves consuming a hearty breakfast, good lunch and a light, early dinner (perhaps soup or vegetables). This can either be done every day or on alternate days.

But remember, what is more important is the quality of food that is consumed. Fasting is no substitute for a healthy diet.

FASTING MADE EASY

There's no need to count calories, which is difficult and time consuming, when you're fasting. If you eat non-starchy vegetables – salad greens, spinach, eggplant, tomatoes, radishes, carrots, cauliflower, beetroot – and also beans during the fasting period it will help you to feel full and maximise fibre intake, which is great for your gut, but they're also really low in calories. You can also add a dressing of a little extra-virgin olive oil, lemon or vinegar, and spices.

One of our studies has shown that even if you eat huge plates of non-starchy vegetables for lunch and dinner twice a week, it's still likely you'll reduce your weekly calorie consumption by about 20 per cent.

SNACK ATTACK

Plenty of eating plans recommend regular snacks, but they aren't necessary. People snack, often on highly processed foods, even when they aren't hungry. It's not something our ancestors were able to do, even as little as a century ago.

Being a little bit hungry is actually a positive sign of health. It indicates the presence of a hormone called ghrelin, which has been shown to inhibit inflammation.

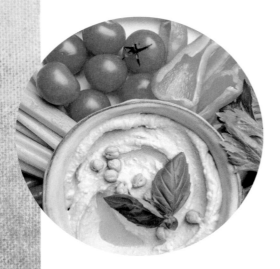

TAKE IT SLOW

A common trait of thin people is that they take their time over a meal – they take a bite and chew it thoroughly, often putting their knife and fork down between mouthfuls. Eating slowly helps a person recognise when they've had enough. People who scoff down their meals consume a large number of calories before they even realise they're full.

To master the art of slow eating, turn off the TV or computer screen so you can focus on the flavour and texture of your food. Choose foods that are high in fibre then chew every mouthful until what you're eating is almost a liquid. Put your fork down each time you take a bite, and talk to your family or friends before you take another.

LEAVE EARLY

In Japan there's a Confucian saying: 'Hara hachi bun me.' It means 'Eat until you are eight out of ten parts full.' Eating from a smaller plate and finishing your meal before you feel full is a very simple way of reducing your calorie intake by about 20 per cent without even trying.

THE MODERN LONGEVITY DIET

My grandmother is from a small village called Mandatoriccio, overlooking the Mediterranean Sea on the east coast of Calabria. She told me stories about what they used to eat. Bread and pasta were made using freshly ground and unrefined local durum wheat. Sourdough starter that was nurtured with love was used to make the dough for the bread.

Grandma Faustina would use tomatoes, eggplant, wild fennel, garlic, hot peppers, herbs and extra-virgin olive oil to top a slice of bread or pizza dough.

Pasta sauce was made with chickpeas, lentils and fava beans. Loads of fresh vegetables were always part of every meal. Salads were created with a mixture of greens – some grown, others foraged – carrots, pumpkins, capers, olives and dressing prepared with extra-virgin olive oil and lemon. Home-cured fish like anchovies and sardines and preserved vegetables were used year round.

One glass of red wine was enjoyed with dinner. Fruit, either fresh or sun-dried, was eaten as a dessert. Meat, fish, milk, cheese and eggs were considered a luxury.

This is the basis of the traditional Mediterranean diet, and people who follow it have low cholesterol, blood pressure and inflammation, healthy guts and a remarkably low incidence of heart disease. People who eat this way often live very long and healthy lives.

I've taken the Mediterranean diet as the basis for my modern healthy longevity diet, although with some modifications. If we were to eat the same amount of olive oil, bread and pasta as my grandparents, for example, we'd undoubtedly gain unhealthy amounts of weight.

> I've taken the Mediterranean diet as the basis for my modern healthy longevity diet.

QUALITY IS KEY

There is no doubt that consuming appropriate amounts of calories and proteins is key for longevity, but it is the quality of our food that will maximise health. Reducing calories while eating unhealthy foods might lead to weight loss, but it can also cause vitamin, mineral and other micro-nutrient deficiencies and even malnutrition.

Our diets need to contain all the essential nutrients our bodies need. Do that by eliminating processed and refined food from your diet and replacing it with a combination of mainly plant-based foods that have a high nutritional value.

Your choices should be diverse, especially when it comes to vegetables, beans and whole grains. They all contain different vitamins, phytochemicals and antioxidants, and eating a variety will ensure you get as many nutrients as possible.

Many people talk about moderation and eating a little bit of everything. But for maximum longevity, 'everything in moderation' is not a dietary rule you should follow. Optimal health is best achieved by cutting out processed foods, refined grains and sugar-sweetened drinks. You need to fill your bank with the freshest and most nutritionally dense food you can find.

THE NEW FOOD PYRAMID

The base of our new pyramid is made up of the foods you should eat every day and consume in the greatest quantities.

For longevity, the base of the pyramid is made up of a wide variety of colourful vegetables, beans, minimally processed whole grains, nuts, seeds and fruits.

Extra-virgin cold-pressed olive oil and avocado should also be consumed daily as condiments, as should spices, lemon juice, or vinegar if you like, and very small amounts of iodised salt.

Two to three times a week you can add fish and shellfish to your meals.

Small portions of cheese and a few free-range organic eggs can be eaten once or twice each week.

Meat and sweets should only be eaten occasionally.

Spring water and herbal teas are the best drinks for staying hydrated.

All sugary and processed drinks, including sodas and juices, should be eliminated from your diet, as should highly processed and refined foods.

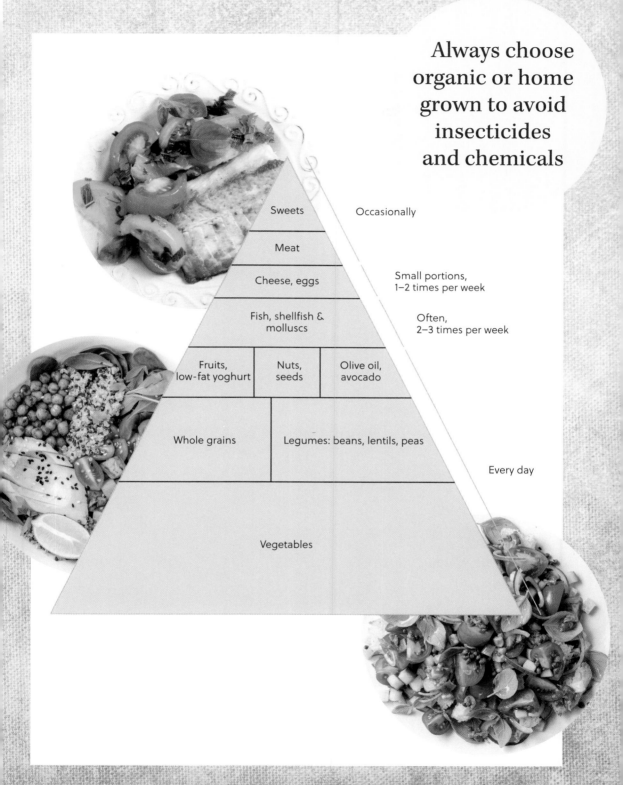

Always choose organic or home grown to avoid insecticides and chemicals

Sweets	Occasionally
Meat	
Cheese, eggs	Small portions, 1–2 times per week
Fish, shellfish & molluscs	Often, 2–3 times per week
Fruits, low-fat yoghurt / Nuts, seeds / Olive oil, avocado	
Whole grains / Legumes: beans, lentils, peas	Every day
Vegetables	

VEGETABLES REAP THE GREATEST REWARD

The word 'vegetable' comes from the Latin *vegetabilis*, which means growing or flourishing. I mention this because vegetables are essential for your ongoing health – they nourish your organs, tissues and cells.

Leafy green, purple and yellow-orange vegetables have the lowest caloric density but the highest concentration of healthy vitamins, minerals and oligoelements (trace elements). Because of their high fibre and water content, these non-starchy vegetables are also essential for maintaining a healthy body weight. In fact, research has proven the higher the intake of vegetables, the better the reduction in body weight and the healthier our gut microbiome.

Counting calories is difficult and takes a lot of time, so creating meals that have a good variety of non-starchy, organic, raw and cooked vegetables – leafy greens, cabbage, carrots, capsicums, pumpkin, avocado, onions – is an excellent way to lower calories while providing your body with huge deposits of vitamins, minerals, oligoelements and other essential nutrients.

One of the keys to making the most of what vegetables have to offer is breaking away from your typical choices, which, for many people, consist of potatoes, lettuce, tomatoes, carrots and perhaps some broccoli.

There are 40 botanical families of vegetables, each one containing hundreds of different varieties. Discovering them, learning how to prepare them and including some in every single meal – both raw and cooked – will add a huge nutritional boost to your diet. Make sure you eat the rainbow.

Consuming white potatoes daily puts people at a higher risk of developing type 2 diabetes. Keep them to once a week, and not fried.

ENERGY? FIBRE? PROTEIN?: GRAINS AND BEANS

As the new food pyramid shows, legumes (beans, lentils and peas) and whole grains should be part of your diet every day. They have many benefits, including reducing glucose levels after a meal during which they're consumed (and after subsequent meals). This benefit is lost, however, if grains are highly milled into flour or prepared at high temperatures. Eating beans, or what some call pulses, at lunch will lower your glycaemic index levels during dinner, too. Consume them during dinner and your night-long glucose levels will remain low. This is extremely important for anyone with prediabetes or diabetes.

Legumes have long been a staple dietary inclusion for many populations, including the centenarians living in Mediterranean countries.

Most beans (except soya beans) are naturally low in fat and are practically free of saturated fatty acids and cholesterol. And while they do contain proteins, they are incomplete. Combine them with whole grains, however, and all nine essential amino acids are obtained in a healthy balance.

Don't be fooled into thinking the more the better. Whole grains do contain high levels of calories. For anyone involved in manual labour or hard exercise, they provide essential amino acids and energy to replenish glycogen stores. If you live a fairly sedentary lifestyle, they're still important – just in lesser quantities. And they're excellent for those who are overweight or obese, particularly those at risk of diabetes, because they're slowly digested and have a relatively low glycaemic index. That means they don't raise blood glucose or insulin levels like many other foods.

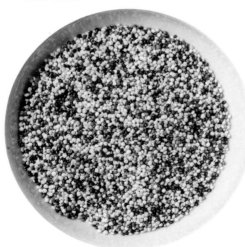

SO EASY TO HAVE ON HAND

There is a misconception that legumes and whole grains are hard
to prepare. That is completely wrong. They're a great product to keep in
your pantry. Keep several varieties on hand – they last for several months
if stored in a dark, cool spot.

The easiest way to make sure you have them ready to add to meals
is to prepare them once or twice a week – two or more different varieties
is a good idea – and store them in the fridge until you need them.

Large pulses, such as chickpeas and fava and borlotti beans,
should be soaked for 24 hours before cooking.

Whenever you're cooking, you can add a cup or two of dried beans, chickpeas
or lentils to a saucepan and simmer them until done. Use at least three cups of
water for every cup of beans since they are nature's little sponges. Keep an eye
on water levels as they're cooking and skim off any foam that rises.

Drain the beans and, once cooled, add a little salt and store them in the fridge
ready for use. This also works for grains like brown rice, farro and barley. These
cooked grains and legumes can easily be added to salads and soups at meal
times. If you're using them in salads, a bit of lemon juice improves the taste
and the availability of vitamins and minerals, especially calcium and iron.

NUTS AND SEEDS

These nutritional powerhouses are often overlooked, but should be included in your daily diet. They provide essential amino acids, fatty acids, dietary fibre and a wide variety of vitamins and oligoelements.

Many people aren't sure how to include them in meals, but they add texture to salads (don't forget about pine nuts) and flavour to sauces, dips and smoothies.

They're a great snack for kids, and I like to take a small bag of nuts (always organic) with me when I travel.

You do need to shop for them with care. The best to buy are organic, raw nuts still in their shells. Some seeds are best soaked overnight before consuming.

There's growing scientific evidence that those who consume a serving of nuts five times a week experience a 40 to 60 per cent lower risk of developing heart disease.

HOW MUCH IS A SERVE OF NUTS?

One serve, or about a handful, of nuts every day is great for your health.
Here are some common varieties and what constitutes a serving.

- 20 almonds
- 9 walnuts
- 15 pecans

- 20 hazelnuts
- 30 pistachio nuts
- 15 cashew nuts

- 2 tablespoons pine nuts

THE IMPORTANCE OF FISH

Japanese and Inuit populations are known for having low rates of heart disease and their common factor is regular fish consumption. Studies show that people who eat certain types of fish – salmon, sardines, herring, mackerel, anchovies, tuna – rich in long-chain omega-3 fatty acids two to four times a week are significantly less likely to have a heart attack than someone who only eats them once a month.

There are other benefits too, from lower risk of stroke to providing high levels of vitamin B12, iron and zinc.

Of course, the fish has to be prepared correctly. Steamed or baked fish is perfect; fried fish provides none of these benefits and may, in fact, if it is fried in oils with trans-fats, increase the risk of ill health.

SWEET RELIEF: FRUIT

Fruit is often excluded from dietary plans. People say it is too full of sugar to be good for you. That's not true. In fact, they're rich in other properties that make them great for your health and skin.

For anyone used to having dessert, fruit is an excellent alternative. Not only is it far lower in calories and fat than cake or ice-cream, but a cup of strawberries or blueberries will be packed with vitamin C. Mango, for example, has vitamin A, vitamin C and vitamin E.

The dietary fibre provided by fruit also forms a gel-like substance that improves gut health and helps you to feel full for longer.

BEST FOODS FOR HEALTHY GLOWING SKIN

Vitamin C, quercetin, anthocyanins: oranges, lemons, blueberries, blackcurrants, strawberries, kiwi fruit, papaya, apples

Antioxidants: carrots, sweet potatoes, pumpkin, broccoli, butter lettuce, parsley, spinach, watercress

Omega-3: oily fish, nuts, seeds, avocado

Phytochemicals: green and herbal tea

THE GOOD OIL

Extra-virgin olive oil is one of the healthiest and most nutritionally balanced condiments. It has been used by Mediterranean populations for centuries. When you're shopping for it, seek out first cold-pressed extra-virgin olive oil, which is a better quality and has a nicer flavour. Check the harvest and bottle date, too. It should be consumed between 12 and 14 months after production.

I use it for dressing salads, raw and cooked vegetables, legumes and pasta sauces. Remember, however, that each tablespoon of olive oil contains 120 calories, so consuming too much can cause weight gain.

ALL-NATURAL FLAVOURS

Humans have used onion, garlic, herbs and spices to add flavour, aroma and colour to food for millennia. Of course, we still appreciate them for all these things, but they also play an important role in making our food more enjoyable while reducing less healthy ingredients such as salt, sugar, butter and vegetable oils.

Culinary herbs and spices contain high concentrations of unique phytochemicals that can provide positive clinical effects – turmeric, for instance, has anti-inflammatory and antioxidant properties, while fresh rosemary contains compounds with possible antioxidant, central nervous system and liver-protective properties – but they also simply transform so-so dishes into something delicious.

WHAT SHOULD I DRINK?

The best way to quench a thirst is with spring water.

The only real improvement on plain water is boiling it and pouring it over tea leaves or herbal infusions, which contain a range of powerful bioactive compounds.

Green, sage and rosemary teas are a year-round favourite. Peppermint tea, especially when chilled, is refreshing during summer. During winter, thyme, ginger and cloves is a warming blend.

Many people get great pleasure and comfort from a cup of black tea. If you do, you should continue to, although don't forget it contains caffeine, which can affect your quality of sleep if too much is consumed.

A PANTRY RESET

In the average Western diet, about 60 per cent of calories come from highly processed foods. The problem is that these are major contributors to the pandemic of obesity, type 2 diabetes, cardiovascular disease, cancer and other life-shortening diseases.

Eliminating or at least significantly decreasing the amount of these industrial foods you consume will overwhelmingly improve your health and longevity.

Any food that has been ultra-processed usually contains high levels of saturated fat, trans-fat and added sugar. Most will also include preservatives and additives that could well have potential carcinogenic actions. Very few will have any vegetable fibre, vitamins or minerals.

These are the foods you should eliminate from your diet:

- soft drinks, even diet ones
- packaged breads and buns
- packaged snacks
- industrialised desserts and cakes
- reconstituted meat products like chicken nuggets and meat balls
- instant noodles and soups
- frozen or shelf-stable ready meals
- any foods made mainly from sugar, oils and fat
- confectionery

RID YOURSELF OF TEMPTATION

If your pantry is stocked with foods that aren't in our new food pyramid, you need to give it a good clean out. You don't need boxes of breakfast cereal, muesli bars, dried fruit, tinned soup, ready-made meals, cordials or anything else that's processed. Your family might object at first, but as you start to explore ways to create tasty meals with food from the pyramid, they'll soon forget they ever snacked on bags of chips.

WHAT ABOUT MEAT?

Western diets are high in meat – beef, lamb, pork, chicken and turkey. Meat is often eaten every day, sometimes even several times a day. Growing evidence, however, suggests that red meat should be limited to between 350 and 500 grams each week. That equates to a medium fillet steak.

The total protein in a typical Western diet is on average at least 40 per cent higher than it needs to be. Excessive meat consumption is implicated in cardiovascular disease, obesity, type 2 diabetes and cancer. Cutting back on animal protein and substituting meat with plant protein has been shown to enhance the capacity of the immune system to destroy malignant cancer cells.

As for processed meats, like bacon, salami, hot dogs and deli meats, these should be removed from your diet as much as possible.

If you're not ready to commit to removing meat completely from your diet, cutting right back can have a number of health benefits, including decreasing your risk of colon cancer and cardiovascular disease. By also choosing ethically sourced animal products you will benefit the welfare of animals and the health of the planet.

Ask yourself:
Do I really need to eat meat today? Did the meat come from industrial farming? Is it good for my health?

SALT

By removing highly processed foods from your diet, you will naturally also eliminate much of the unnecessary sodium. A small amount of salt is important for many biological functions, but you should choose iodised salt for daily use. Limit it to about half a teaspoon each day to be used in cooking and seasoning. This won't give you the necessary daily amount of iodine, so add dried seaweeds, marine seafood or small amounts of cheese or milk to your diet to supplement it.

SUPPLEMENTS

Speaking of supplements, you shouldn't rely on them to provide you with extra vitamins and minerals. Supplements cannot replace all the complex but balanced array of vitamins, phytochemicals, minerals and elements contained in whole foods. And they are no replacement for a healthy, well-balanced diet, unless prescribed by your doctor for a specific health condition.

There is no doubt in my mind that consuming the appropriate amounts of calories and proteins is the most important factor in promoting health and longevity, but the quality of these calories and proteins is key.

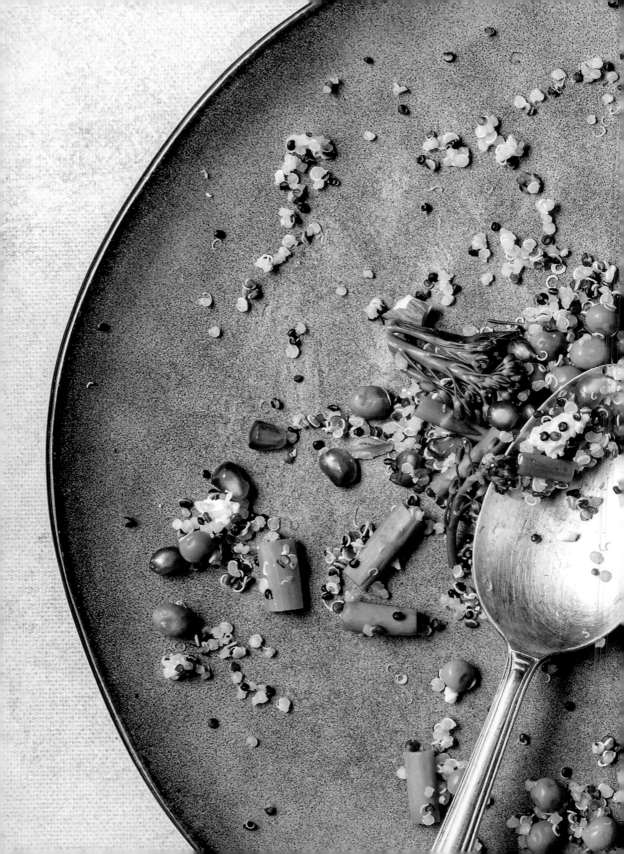

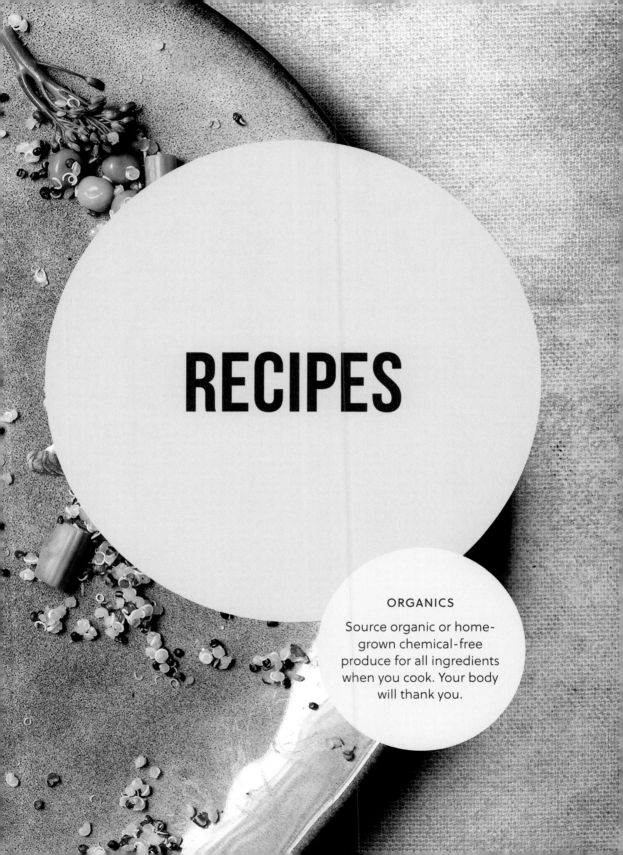

RECIPES

ORGANICS

Source organic or home-grown chemical-free produce for all ingredients when you cook. Your body will thank you.

BREAKFAST

CHIA PUDDING
WITH CINNAMON, BANANA AND NUTS

SERVES 1 • PREPARATION TIME **SOAKING OVERNIGHT, THEN 5 MINUTES**

2 tablespoons chia seeds

3 tablespoons almond milk

1 vanilla bean, split lengthways and seeds scraped

1½ teaspoons honey

½ banana, thinly sliced

2 tablespoons roughly chopped almonds

pinch of ground cinnamon

Chia seeds can be easily added to a morning fruit smoothie or to a bean soup for extra texture and nutrition. Recent studies have shown them to be one of the richest plant sources of omega-3 fatty acids. They are also a rich source of calcium, phosphorus, zinc and copper. Several studies suggest a potential protective effect of chia seeds in reducing cholesterol and body weight.

Eating chia pudding is a great way to feel full while enjoying a breakfast that is nutrient-rich.

Combine the chia seeds, almond milk, vanilla seeds (keep the vanilla bean for another use), 1 teaspoon honey and 100 ml (3½ fl oz) water in an airtight container and leave to soak overnight in the refrigerator.

To serve, spoon the chia mixture into a glass or bowl and top with the banana and chopped almonds. Drizzle over the remaining honey and sprinkle with cinnamon.

VARIATIONS

Replace the banana and cinnamon with half a mango and 1 teaspoon flaked dried coconut for a tropical twist. Or sprinkle with goji berries and coconut.

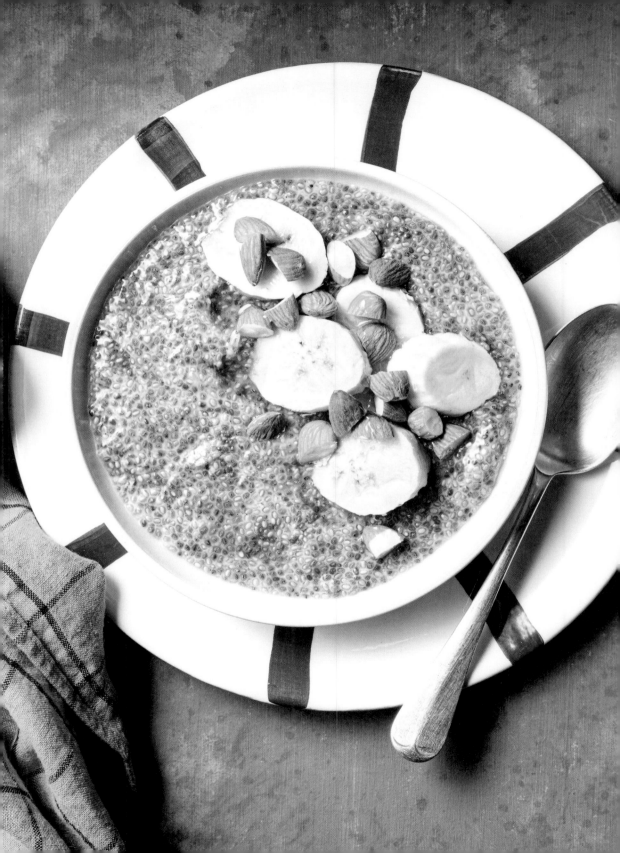

OAT AND HAZELNUT PORRIDGE

SERVES **4** • PREPARATION TIME **5 MINUTES** • COOKING TIME **15 MINUTES**

50 g (1¾ oz) steel-cut oats

200 ml (7 fl oz) almond milk

100 g (3½ oz/⅔ cup) fresh or frozen blueberries

1 teaspoon Dutch (unsweetened) cocoa powder

2 tablespoons chopped hazelnuts

Hazelnuts are an excellent source of vitamin E and are rich in fibre, folate and potassium. Hazelnuts are also one of the richest sources of proanthocyanidins, which seem to play a role in lowering lipid free radicals.

Oats are both filling and slow to break down in your gut, giving you a full feeling while the nutrients slowly release.

Put the oats in a saucepan then stir in the almond milk and 240 ml (8 fl oz) water. Bring to the boil, then reduce the heat and simmer gently for 10–15 minutes, stirring occasionally, or until creamy.

Spoon the porridge into serving bowls and top with blueberries. Sprinkle over the cocoa powder and hazelnuts.

MULTIGRAIN PORRIDGE
WITH PEAR AND PISTACHIO NUTS

SERVES 2 • PREPARATION TIME **SOAKING OVERNIGHT, THEN 5 MINUTES**
COOKING TIME **15 MINUTES**

1 tablespoon millet

1 tablespoon
  amaranth

1 tablespoon
  buckwheat groats

1 tablespoon quinoa

200 ml (7 fl oz) oat
  milk, plus extra
  if desired

1 ripe pear, peeled
  and cored

1 tablespoon
  pistachio nuts,
  chopped

2 medjool dates,
  pitted and sliced

ground cinnamon, for
  dusting (optional)

A good source of protein and potassium, pistachio nuts contain higher carotenoids and chlorophylls than other tree nuts. They also have appreciable amounts of polyphenol stilbenes, which seem to promote anti-cancer, anti-inflammatory and antioxidant activities.

Mix the grains in a bowl and cover with water. Leave to soak overnight, then drain and rinse well.

Place the grains in a saucepan with the oat milk. Bring to the boil, then turn down the heat and simmer gently for 15 minutes. Stir occasionally, until most of the oat milk is absorbed and the grains are soft. Add more oat milk if it is too thick for your liking.

Spoon the porridge into two serving bowls. Mash half the pear with a fork and stir through the porridge. Dice the other half of the pear and put on top. Sprinkle with pistachio nuts and sliced dates. Dust with cinnamon if desired.

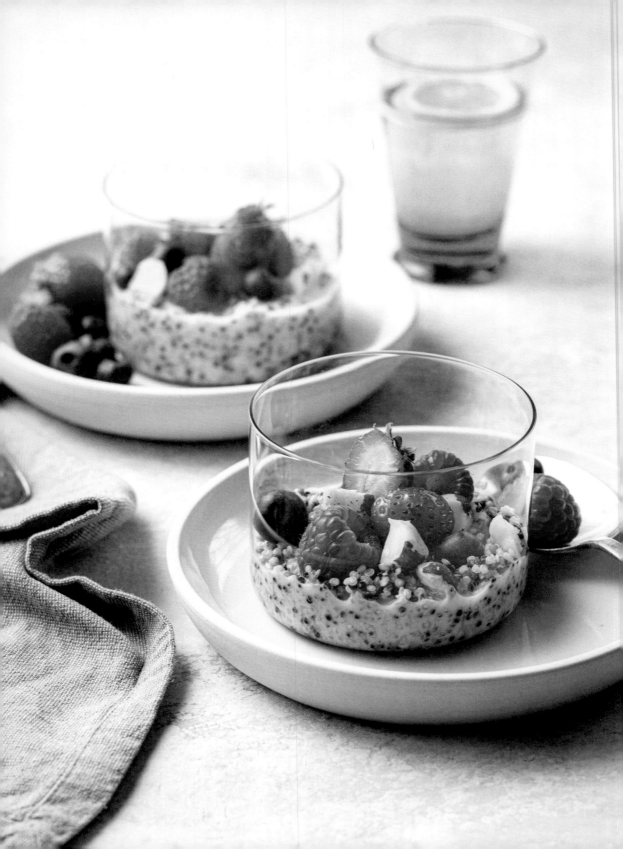

QUINOA PORRIDGE
WITH BERRIES AND BRAZIL NUTS

SERVES **2** · PREPARATION TIME **5 MINUTES** · COOKING TIME **15 MINUTES**

250 ml (8½ fl oz/1 cup) almond milk, plus extra if desired

100 g (3½ oz/½ cup) quinoa, rinsed

1 teaspoon honey

3 tablespoons fresh or frozen mixed berries

1 tablespoon roughly chopped Brazil nuts

Quinoa is a great source of carbohydrate and protein. By adding both berries and Brazil nuts (rich in the powerful antioxidant selenium), you will get fantastic nutrients as well. You can freeze this porridge for a ready-made breakfast.

Warm two-thirds of the almond milk in a saucepan over a medium heat, then add the quinoa, stirring well. Bring to a simmer and cook for about 15 minutes, stirring, or until all the liquid has been absorbed.

Remove the porridge from the heat and stir in the honey and berries, then divide between bowls. Scatter over the chopped nuts and pour an extra 2–3 tablespoons of almond milk over each bowl if you prefer a thinner consistency for your porridge. Serve.

VARIATIONS

You can swap out half the berries for half a small banana, and replace the Brazil nuts with walnuts or pecans, if you prefer.

BREAKFAST BRUSCHETTA WITH TOMATO AND FETA

SERVES **2** · PREPARATION TIME **10 MINUTES** · COOKING TIME **15 MINUTES**

2 slices sourdough
bread

2 tomatoes, sliced

20 g (¾ oz) feta,
crumbled

2 free-range eggs

freshly ground black
pepper

1 handful torn basil
leaves

1 handful baby rocket
(arugula)

This is a pizza-inspired bruschetta, but a lot healthier. Sourdough aids digestion and the flavour of tomato, feta and basil is always delicious.

Preheat the oven to 180°C (350°F).

Toast the bread and place the slices on a baking tray.

Arrange the sliced tomatoes on top of the bread. Scatter the feta over the tomatoes. Crack an egg on top of each slice, then season with pepper (no need for salt when you are using feta).

Bake for 10–15 minutes, or until the egg is cooked to your liking. Sprinkle with fresh basil leaves and rocket.

SOURDOUGH TOAST
WITH PEANUT CREAM AND FRUIT TOPPING

SERVES **4** • PREPARATION TIME **10 MINUTES**

4 slices sourdough
  bread

100 g (3½ oz/⅔ cup)
  blueberries

2 peaches, stoned
  and thinly sliced

12 almonds, chopped

PEANUT CREAM

100 g (3½ oz) peanuts

1 Brazil nut

1 tablespoon lemon
  juice

Peanuts are actually legumes, and they are rich in folate, which plays a key role in DNA synthesis and repair, and in brain development.

To prepare the peanut cream, combine the ingredients in a food processor and blend until combined. Add about 1 tablespoon of water to achieve a creamy consistency like peanut butter. You might need to stop the blender occasionally to push the mixture down with a spatula.

Toast the bread and spread with a thin layer of the peanut cream. For each slice, cover half with blueberries and the other half with peach slices. Sprinkle with almonds.

VARIATIONS

You can swap out peanut cream and replace it with any nut butter and replace the peaches and blueberries with bananas, plums – any of your favourites.

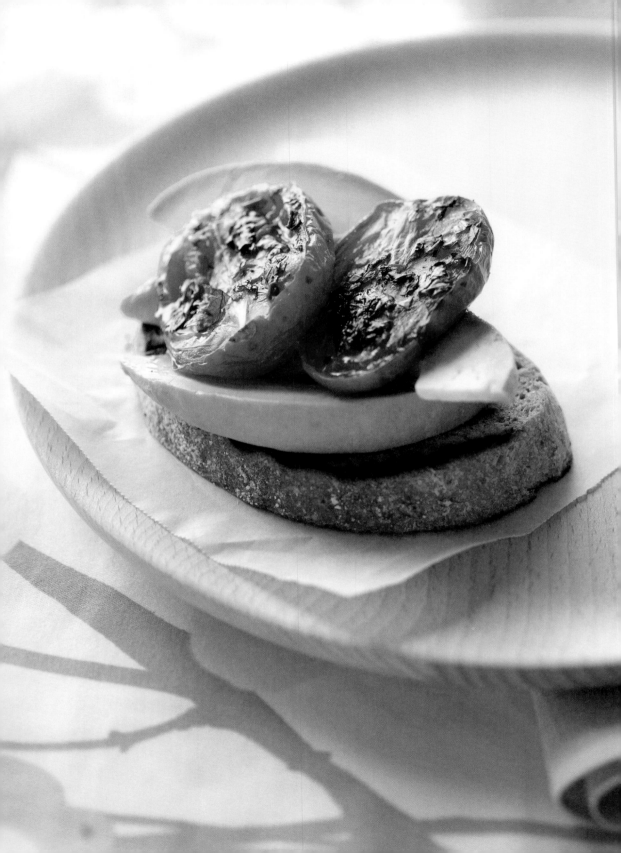

BRUSCHETTA WITH TOMATO AND AVOCADO

SERVES 1
PREPARATION TIME **5 MINUTES**
COOKING TIME **5 MINUTES**

1 teaspoon extra-virgin olive oil

1 tomato, halved

2 or 3 basil leaves (or parsley leaves), finely chopped

1 slice sourdough rye bread

½ avocado, peeled, stone removed and sliced

salt and freshly ground black pepper

A perfect light and healthy breakfast.

Heat the oil in a small frying pan over a medium heat. Add the two tomato halves, skin side down. Sprinkle the tomatoes with basil. Lower the heat to medium and cook for 2 or 3 minutes or until the tomatoes start to soften.

Meanwhile, toast the rye bread.

To serve, top the toast with the avocado slices, then the tomato halves. Season with salt and pepper.

BRUSCHETTA WITH EGG AND AVOCADO

SERVES 1
PREPARATION TIME **5 MINUTES**
COOKING TIME **5 MINUTES**

1 free-range egg

1 teaspoon finely chopped chives

salt and freshly ground black pepper

½ teaspoon extra-virgin olive oil

1 slice sourdough rye bread

1 handful baby spinach leaves

½ avocado, peeled, stone removed and sliced

Whisk together the egg and chives in a small bowl. Season with salt and pepper.

Heat the oil in a small frying pan over a medium heat. Add the egg mixture and cook for 2–3 minutes, gently pushing it in from the edge until the egg is just cooked.

Meanwhile, toast the rye bread.

To serve, top the toast with the spinach leaves, then the cooked egg and avocado slices. Season with salt and pepper.

PUMPKIN, CAPSICUM AND PESTO BRUSCHETTA

SERVES **2**
PREPARATION TIME **5 MINUTES**
COOKING TIME **3 MINUTES**

200 g (7 oz) pumpkin (winter squash), thinly sliced
1 teaspoon extra-virgin olive oil
2 thyme sprigs
2 slices sourdough bread
1 teaspoon Simple pesto (page 85)
½ red capsicum (bell pepper), seeds removed and finely diced
1 small handful rocket (arugula)

Pumpkin is both dense in nutrients and low in calories, making it a winning combination for breakfast or a light lunch.

Preheat the oven to 180°C (350°F).

Arrange the pumpkin slices on a baking tray, brush with olive oil and sprinkle with fresh thyme leaves. Roast in the oven for 20–25 minutes, or until softened. Set the pumpkin aside to cool slightly.

Toast the bread and spread the pesto evenly over the toast. Pile the pumpkin on top with the capsicum. Finish with the rocket.

TOASTED WHOLEMEAL BREAD WITH MUSHROOMS AND GOAT'S CHEESE

SERVES **2**
PREPARATION TIME **10 MINUTES**
COOKING TIME **20 MINUTES**

1 teaspoon extra-virgin olive oil
½ garlic clove, finely chopped
50 g (1¾ oz) mushrooms, thinly sliced
2 slices wholemeal (whole-wheat) bread
½ avocado, peeled, stone removed and mashed
9 cherry tomatoes, sliced in half and seasoned with salt
50 g (1¾ oz/⅓ cup) goat's cheese

Surprisingly, avocados are higher in potassium – a nutrient most people don't get enough of – than bananas.

Heat the olive oil in a small frying pan over a low–medium heat. Add the garlic and the mushrooms. Sauté for 1–3 minutes.

Meanwhile, toast the bread and spread the slices with a generous layer of the avocado. Top with the sliced mushrooms then the cherry tomatoes. Sprinkle with goat's cheese.

TOASTED WHOLEMEAL BREAD TOPPED WITH HOME-MADE HUMMUS AND RED ONION

SERVES **2** • PREPARATION TIME **10 MINUTES**
COOKING TIME **5 MINUTES**

½ small red onion, peeled and finely sliced into rings

2 large slices wholemeal (whole-wheat) bread

2 tablespoons Home-made hummus (see page 123)

8 ripe cherry tomatoes, diced

1 small cucumber, finely sliced

1 tablespoon extra-virgin olive oil

salt and freshly ground black pepper

dried oregano, to garnish

Almost any salad vegetable could be used to top the hummus and red onion: cucumber, tomato, radish, asparagus, lettuce, capsicum (bell peppers) ... the list is endless.

Half fill a small saucepan with water and bring to a boil. Add the onion rings to the pan and cook for 2 minutes. Drain the onion rings and set aside to cool.

Toast the bread and spread with a generous layer of the hummus. Top the hummus with the onion rings, followed by the cherry tomatoes and cucumber. Drizzle with the extra-virgin olive oil and season with salt and pepper. Garnish with oregano.

VARIATIONS

Replace the cherry tomatoes with sun-dried tomatoes and replace the cucumber with sliced zucchini (courgette) or red capsicum (bell pepper).

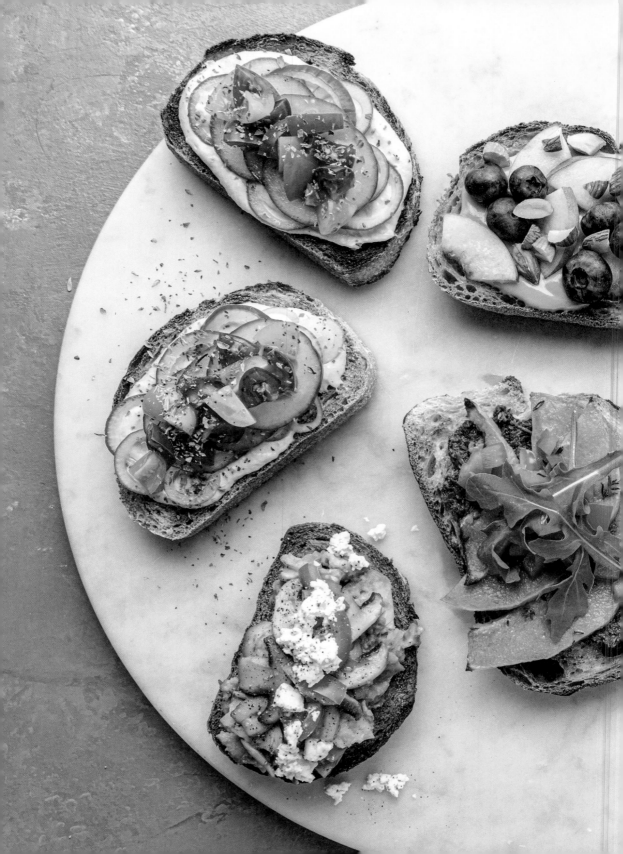

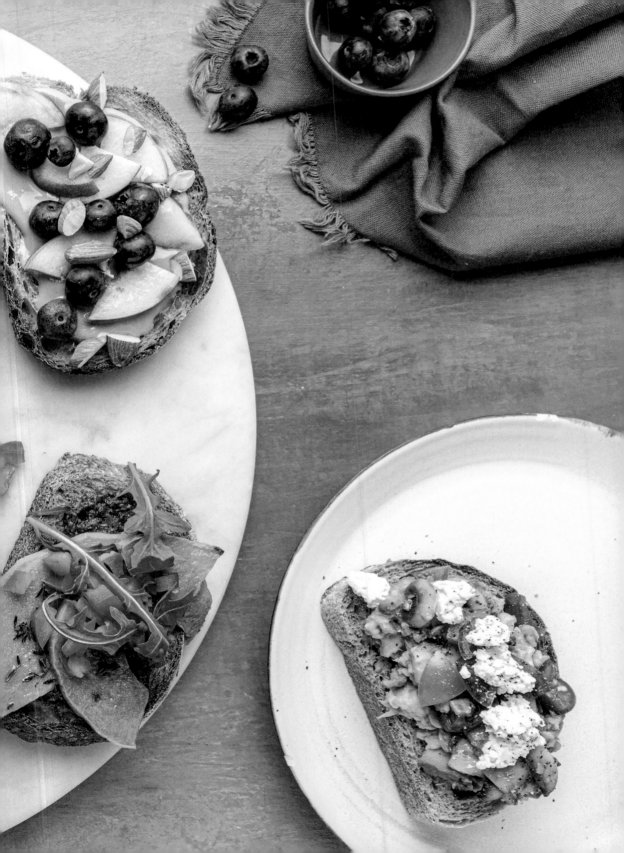

SMOOTHIES & JUICES

BERRY AND ALMOND SMOOTHIE

SERVES **2** • PREPARATION TIME **10 MINUTES**

80 g (2¾ oz/½ cup) frozen blueberries

1 small ripe banana

160 ml (5½ fl oz) almond milk, plus extra if needed

1 small carrot, peeled and roughly chopped

40 ml (1¼ fl oz) freshly squeezed orange juice

10 almonds

2 Brazil nuts

The fruit of a South American tree, Brazil nuts are one of my favourite nuts. They are rich in selenium: just one nut supplies more than the recommended daily amount for selenium, a powerful antioxidant mineral that helps to prevent tissue damage caused by free radicals. Two or three times a week, I add a couple of these nuts, together with a couple of teaspoons of unsweetened dark cocoa powder, to my morning fruit smoothies.

Put all the ingredients in a blender or food processor and blend until well combined. Add a little more almond milk or chilled water until you achieve a creamy consistency that is not too thick.

VARIATIONS

Replace the carrot with 125 g (4½ oz) raw beetroot (beets) and a slice of fresh ginger.

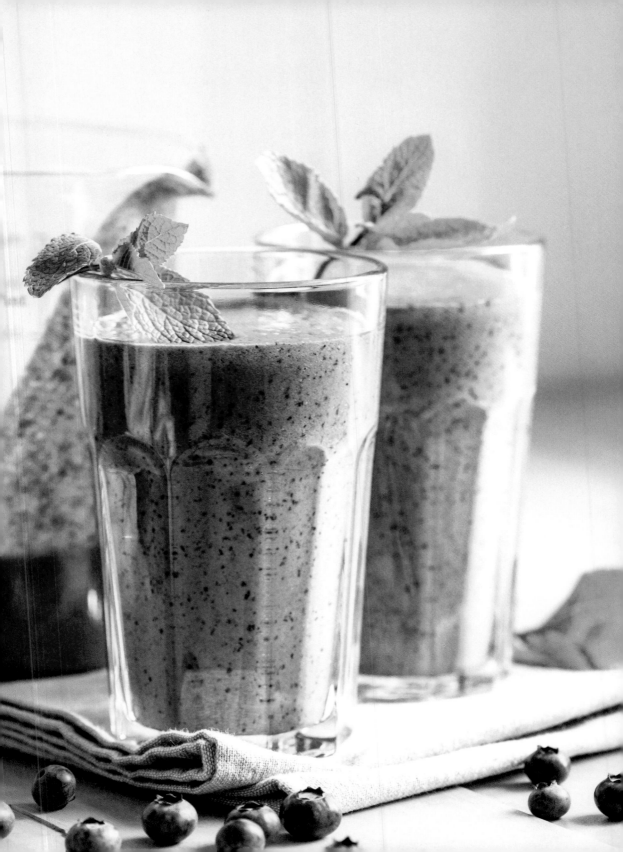

MANGO AND OAT MILK BREAKFAST SMOOTHIE

SERVES **2** · PREPARATION TIME **10 MINUTES**

1 large ripe mango,
  peeled and diced

1 small ripe banana

½ avocado

160 ml (5½ fl oz)
  oat milk, plus extra
  if needed

40 ml (1¼ fl oz)
  freshly squeezed
  orange juice

5 walnuts

2 Brazil nuts

1 medjool date, pitted

TOPPING

20 blueberries

1 tablespoon linseeds
  (flax seeds)

Almonds are a very rich source of the powerful antioxidant vitamin E. A small handful (approximately 30 g/1 oz) provides vitamin E and magnesium, which play a role in lowering blood pressure. They are also a good source of protein and calcium. Home-made almond milk, made from spring water and raw almonds, is a terrific substitute for store-bought almond milk.

Put all the ingredients in a blender or food processor and blend until well combined. Add a little more oat milk or chilled water until you achieve a creamy consistency that is not too thick. Top with blueberries and linseeds.

STRAWBERRY, GINGER AND BEETROOT SMOOTHIE

SERVES **4** • PREPARATION TIME **10 MINUTES**

150 g (5½ oz/1 cup)
  strawberries, hulled

115 g (4 oz/1½ cups)
  cos (romaine)
  lettuce

1 small avocado,
  peeled, stone
  removed and diced

½ red beetroot (beet),
  peeled and diced

125 ml (4 fl oz/½ cup)
  unsweetened
  oat milk

1 cm (½ in) piece
  ginger, peeled and
  roughly sliced

1 tablespoon honey

1 tablespoon linseeds
  (flax seeds)

Also called flax seeds, linseeds are an important source of antioxidant lignans (up to 13 mg per gram) and heart-friendly omega-3 alpha-linolenic acid. After oily fish, linseeds are an excellent source of omega-3 fatty acids in our diet and have been shown to have a small but significant reduction in total and LDL-cholesterol. Because of the high polyunsaturated fat content, it's best to keep the linseeds and their oil in the refrigerator to avoid oxidation.

Place the strawberries, lettuce, avocado and beetroot in a food processor. Add 125 ml (4 fl oz/½ cup) water and the oat milk and blitz at high speed for 1 minute. Then add all the remaining ingredients and keep blending until smooth.

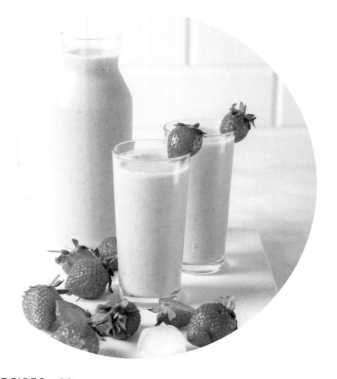

MEDICINAL GREEN JUICE

SERVES 4 • PREPARATION TIME 10 MINUTES

1 large apple, peeled

1 large carrot, peeled

4 large cos (romaine)
  lettuce leaves

4 large silverbeet
  (Swiss chard) leaves

1 large cabbage or
  kale leaf

1 celery stalk

½ red capsicum
  (bell pepper),
  seeds removed

½ red beetroot (beet),
  peeled and diced

1 cm (½ in) piece
  ginger, peeled
  and sliced

This is a quick and convenient way to boost your nutrients and consume a diverse array of vegetables in one hit.

Place all the ingredients, one after the other, in a juice extractor to produce a super-healthy juice. Mix well before drinking.

VARIATIONS

Juices can include all sorts of organic fruits and vegetables and creating your own favourites by experimenting with combinations is a lot of fun.

CUCUMBER, APPLE AND MINT SMOOTHIE

SERVES 4 • PREPARATION TIME 10 MINUTES

1 large cucumber,
 peeled and sliced

1 small avocado,
 peeled, stone
 removed and diced

5 g (⅛ oz/¼ cup) mint
 leaves

125 ml (4 fl oz/½ cup)
 unsweetened
 oat milk

1 green apple, peeled
 and diced

1 tablespoon honey

2 tablespoons
 sunflower kernels

Place the cucumber, avocado and mint in a food processor. Add 125 ml (4 fl oz/½ cup) water and the oat milk and blend at high speed for 1 minute. Then add the apple, honey and sunflower kernels and blend until smooth. Sprinkle with your favourite seeds or nuts to serve.

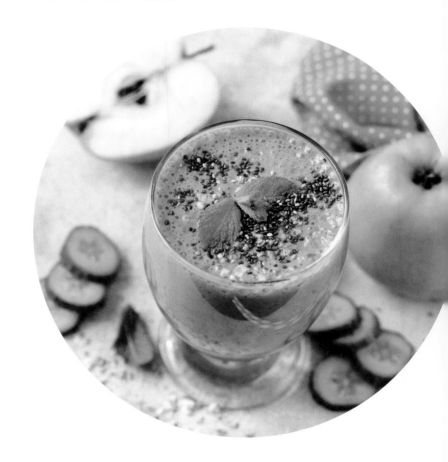

SOUP

RIBOLLITA (A HEARTY TUSCAN WHITE BEAN AND VEGETABLE SOUP)

SERVES **4** · PREPARATION TIME **30 MINUTES** · COOKING TIME **2 HOURS**

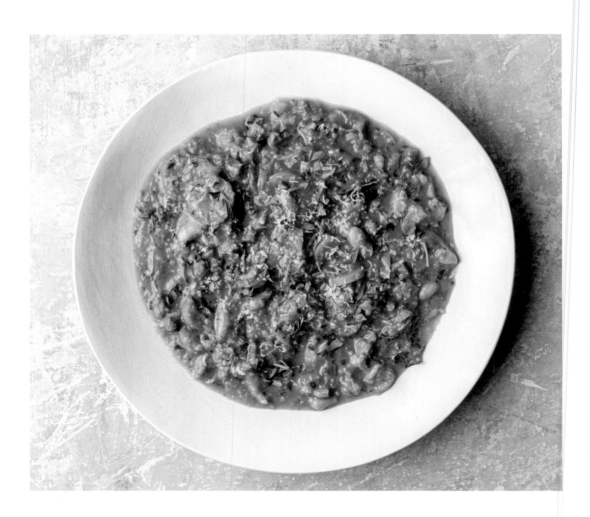

125 g (4½ oz) dried cannellini (lima) beans, soaked in water overnight

2 celery leaves

3–4 thyme sprigs

3–4 rosemary sprigs

100 g (3½ oz) silverbeet (Swiss chard)

250 g (9 oz) white cabbage

250 g (9 oz) purple cabbage

2 tablespoons extra-virgin olive oil, plus extra for drizzling

1 onion, finely chopped

4 garlic cloves, crushed and chopped

1 large carrot, sliced in rounds

1 leek, finely chopped

400 g (14 oz) tomatoes, peeled and diced or crushed

1 parmesan rind (optional), plus extra grated parmesan to serve

1 teaspoon salt

1 teaspoon freshly ground black pepper

¼ teaspoon chilli flakes

30 g (1 oz/1 cup) chopped flat-leaf (Italian) parsley

juice of ½ lemon

4 slices of crusty sourdough bread

Drain the cannellini beans and cook in a medium pot of boiling salted water with a couple of celery leaves until tender (see pages 130–131), about 1–1½ hours. When ready, remove the celery and drain the beans, reserving 500 ml (17 fl oz/2 cups) of the cooking water. Blend one-third of the cannellini beans in a food processor with some of the reserved cooking water. Set aside the puréed beans and the remaining whole beans.

Make a bouquet garni of thyme and rosemary by tying them together in a little bundle with kitchen twine. Set aside.

Separate the stems and leaves of the silverbeet and cabbage with a sharp knife, then chop both but keep the stems separate.

In the meantime, heat the olive oil in a large, heavy-based pot over a medium heat. Add the onion and garlic and sauté for 2 minutes. Reduce the heat to low–medium and add 1 ladle of bean stock together with the carrot, leek and the stems of the silverbeet and cabbage. Cook for another 10 minutes. Add the tomatoes and parmesan rind with the salt, pepper and chilli flakes and continue cooking, stirring occasionally, for 7–8 minutes.

Add the leaves of the silverbeet and cabbage to the soup. Also add the bouquet garni. Add more bean stock, if needed, and cook until the vegetables are tender, then remove the thyme and rosemary, and the parmesan rind, from the pot. Add the bean puree and whole cooked beans. Cook for another 5 minutes so that all the ingredients are mixed well and heated through. Stir in the parsley and lemon juice and pour the hot ribollita into individual bowls.

Top the ribollita with a drizzle of olive oil and sprinkle with grated parmesan. Serve with sourdough bread.

BARLEY, BEAN AND ASPARAGUS SOUP

SERVES **4** • PREPARATION TIME **10 MINUTES** • COOKING TIME **40 MINUTES**

75 g (2¾ oz)
 unpearled barley

1 tablespoon extra-
 virgin olive oil, plus
 4 teaspoons extra to
 serve

1 onion, finely
 chopped

2 garlic cloves, finely
 chopped

1 leek, trimmed and
 finely chopped

750 ml (25½ fl oz/
 3 cups) vegetable
 stock

500 g (1 lb 2 oz)
 asparagus, cut
 into chunks

200 g (7 oz/4 cups)
 baby spinach

400 g (14 oz)
 cannellini (lima)
 beans, cooked (see
 page 130–131)

salt and freshly
 ground black pepper

Wheat, barley and legumes, rather than meat, were the staple foods of gladiators in Ancient Rome, as a study on their bones by the Department of Forensic Medicine at the Medical University of Vienna has demonstrated. Beans and minimally processed whole grains were also the staple foods of populations with many healthy nonagenarians and centenarians. As the food pyramid shows, grains and beans should be consumed daily. Unlike refined carbohydrates, the consumption of minimally processed whole grains and beans are essential for optimal health.

Cook the barley in a small saucepan of boiling water for about 30–40 minutes, or until tender. Drain well.

Heat the olive oil in a large saucepan over a high heat and add onion, garlic and leek. Sauté for 1 minute. Pour in the vegetable stock, then add the asparagus and spinach. Bring to the boil, then reduce the heat to low and allow the soup to simmer for 10 minutes. Then add the pre-cooked cannellini beans and heat through.

Pour into four soup bowls, adding 2–3 tablespoons of barley to each bowl. Stir well. Season with 1 teaspoon of olive oil per bowl, and some salt and pepper.

SPICY RED LENTIL SOUP

SERVES **4** • PREPARATION TIME **10 MINUTES** • COOKING TIME **1 HOUR**

250 g (9 oz/1 cup) red lentils, rinsed

juice of 1 lime

1 teaspoon ground turmeric

1 teaspoon extra-virgin olive oil

1 onion, chopped

4 garlic cloves, crushed

1 teaspoon ground cumin

1 teaspoon ground coriander

¼ teaspoon chilli powder

400 g (14 oz) chopped tomatoes

25 g (1 oz/½ cup) chopped coriander (cilantro)

4 teaspoons low-fat Greek-style yoghurt, to serve

You can make a big batch of soup and have it on hand for a hearty meal that is both filling and nutritious.

Place the rinsed lentils, lime juice and turmeric in a saucepan. Add enough water to cover the lentils by 3 cm (1¼ in). Bring to the boil over a medium heat then simmer gently for 20–30 minutes, or until the lentils are tender. Drain the lentils.

Heat the olive oil in a saucepan over a medium heat. Cook the onion and garlic for 5 minutes, or until the onion is soft. Add the spices and cook for 1 minute, until fragrant. Stir in the tomato and 125 ml (4 fl oz/½ cup) water and simmer for 5 minutes. Add the cooked lentils and a further 250 ml (8½ fl oz/1 cup) water to the tomato mixture. Simmer for 5 minutes, to warm through. When ready to serve, stir in the coriander, ladle into bowls and top each with a teaspoon of yoghurt.

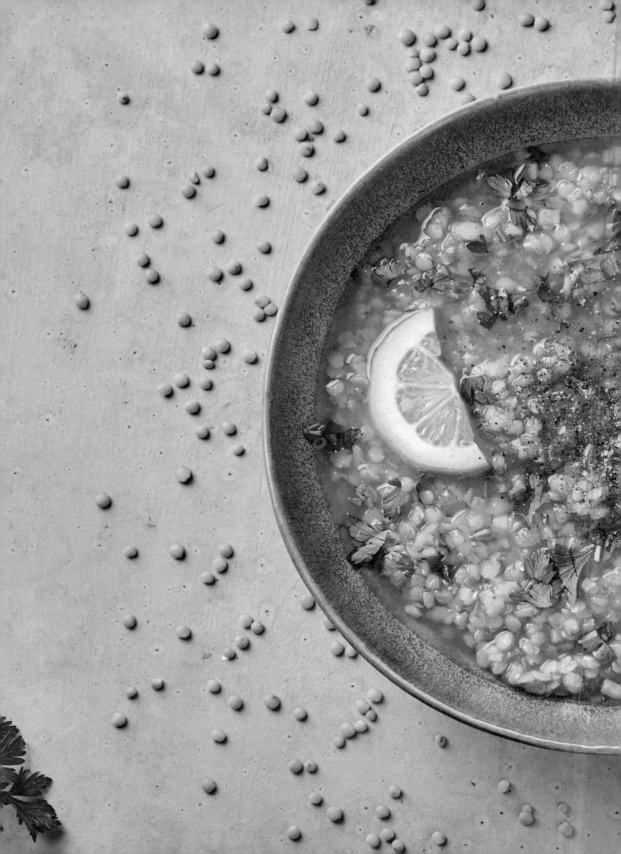

HOT LENTIL SOUP

250 g (9 oz/1 cup) red lentils, rinsed

2 celery leaves

1 teaspoon mustard seeds

1 tablespoon ground coriander

1 tablespoon ground cumin

½ teaspoon ground fenugreek

pinch of salt

1 tablespoon olive oil

2 tablespoons grated ginger

3 green or red chillies, deseeded and finely chopped

4 tomatoes, chopped

juice of ½ lemon

4 teaspoons chopped flat-leaf (Italian) parsley

This soup includes ginger and studies in healthy men and women have shown cooked ginger speeds up gastric emptying, promotes satiety and increases the heat-producing (thermic) effect of food – all factors that can help in the prevention of obesity.

Place the rinsed lentils and celery in a saucepan. Add enough water to cover the lentils by 3 cm (1¼ in). Bring to the boil over a medium heat then simmer gently for 20–30 minutes, or until the lentils are tender. Remove the celery. Drain the lentils, reserving 250 ml (8½ fl oz/1 cup) of the cooking water.

Place the mustard seeds, coriander, cumin, fenugreek and salt in a mortar, or in a small food processor, and grind finely.

Heat the olive oil in a frying pan over a medium heat and add the ground spices. Leave for only a minute or two until the spices begin to give off their aroma, then add the ginger, chilli and tomato. Sauté well until the tomatoes are well cooked, then add the reserved cooking water and simmer for about 6 minutes.

Add the cooked lentils and salt to taste, stirring well. Just before serving add the lemon juice and the parsley and mix well.

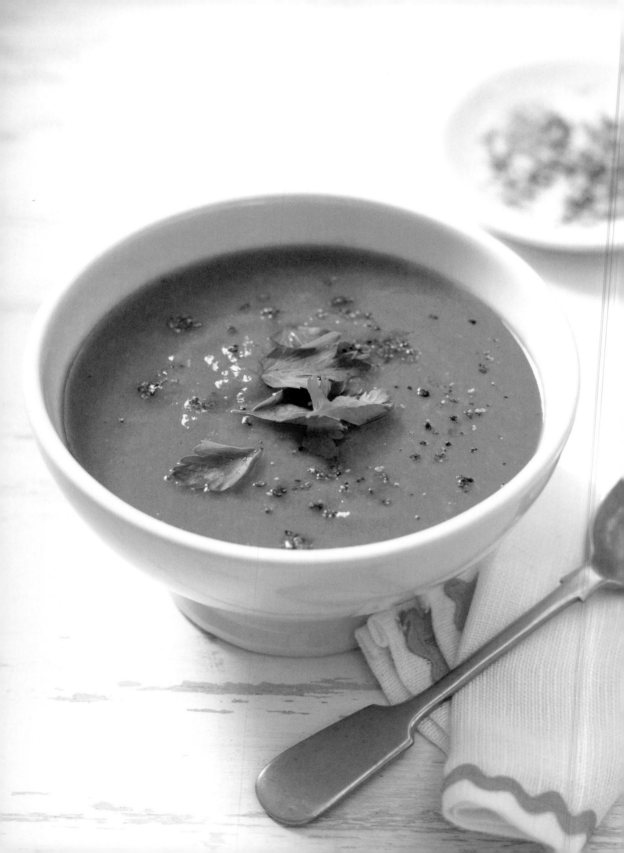

ROASTED TOMATO AND RED CAPSICUM SOUP

SERVES **4** · PREPARATION TIME **20 MINUTES** · COOKING TIME **1 HOUR 20 MINUTES**

800 g (1 lb 12 oz)
  tomatoes, halved

2 red capsicums
  (bell peppers)

1 teaspoon extra-
  virgin olive oil

1 onion, chopped

1 teaspoon smoked
  paprika

1 potato, chopped

750 ml (25½ fl oz/
  3 cups) vegetable
  stock

parsley, to serve

4 teaspoons
  low-fat Greek-style
  yoghurt, to serve
  (optional)

Roasting the tomatoes and capsicum (bell pepper) first concentrates their flavour and sweetness.

Preheat the oven to 220°C (430°F). Place the tomatoes and capsicums on a baking tray and bake for 30 minutes, or until the capsicum skins are wrinkled and the tomatoes have collapsed.

Place the capsicums in a paper bag and leave to cool completely. Set the tomatoes aside to cool. Peel and discard the skins from both the tomatoes and capsicums. Also discard the capsicum seeds.

Heat the oil in a large saucepan over a medium heat. Cook the onion for 5 minutes, stirring occasionally, until soft. Add the paprika and stir for 1 minute, until fragrant. Add the roasted tomatoes and capsicums to the pan with the potato and stock and bring to the boil. Reduce the heat to low and simmer for 30 minutes. Purée with a hand-held blender. Reheat gently over a low heat.

Ladle into bowls and serve each topped with parsley and a teaspoon of yoghurt if desired.

SALADS

ITALIAN ORANGE AND FENNEL SALAD

SERVES **4** • PREPARATION TIME **10 MINUTES**

3 large oranges

1 large fennel bulb, trimmed and thinly sliced (reserve any fronds for serving)

3 tablespoons extra-virgin olive oil

salt and freshly ground black pepper

2 handfuls rocket (arugula), optional

We all know that vegetables are good for us. They are packed with fibre, vitamins and minerals and, importantly, they also have the bulk that we need to feel full and satisfied.

We should be eating two to three serves of vegetables or salad every day. And most vegetables have very low calories, which means you can eat as much as you like without worrying about gaining weight.

Peel two of the oranges and slice them with a sharp knife, or segment them. Place in a bowl with the fennel.

Juice the third orange.

In a small bowl, whisk together the orange juice, olive oil and some salt and pepper, then pour it over the salad. Toss to combine.

Garnish with fresh fennel fronds and rocket if using.

VARIATIONS

Replace oranges with grapefruit segments and add mint to the salad.

ORANGE, RADISH AND MINT SALAD

SERVES 4 • **PREPARATION TIME 10 MINUTES**

4 oranges, peeled and sliced

8 radishes, thinly sliced

½ red onion, thinly sliced

½ fennel bulb, trimmed and finely sliced

3 tablespoons extra-virgin olive oil

pinch of salt

2 mint leaves, finely chopped

4 almonds, finely chopped

Mix the orange, radish, onion and fennel in a serving bowl, then add the olive oil and salt. Toss to combine, then sprinkle with mint and nuts.

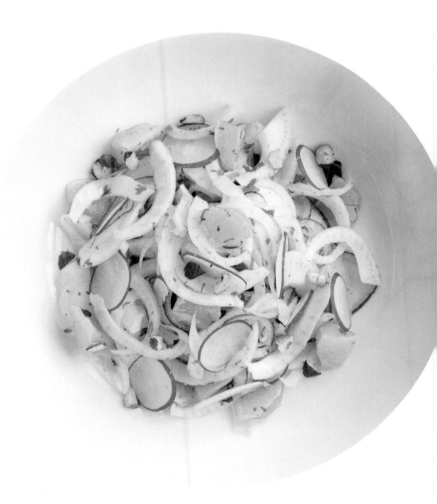

ANCIENT ROMAN COLUMELLA SALAD WITH ALMONDS

SERVES 4 · PREPARATION TIME 10 MINUTES

120 g (4½ oz) rocket (arugula)

120 g (4½ oz) curly endive leaves

2 spring onions (scallions) or 1 small leek, sliced

3 kale or chicory (endive) leaves, stems discarded

10 mint leaves, chopped

2 tablespoons chopped flat-leaf (Italian) parsley

1 teaspoon chopped coriander (cilantro)

1 teaspoon chopped savory (optional)

1 teaspoon thyme leaves

75 g (2¾ oz/½ cup) salted ricotta, crumbled

1 tablespoon white-wine vinegar

salt and freshly ground black pepper

1 tablespoon extra-virgin olive oil

10 almonds, coarsely chopped

olives and toasted sourdough bread, to serve

The ancient Romans used many wild plants in this salad. The diversity of the plants provided a wide range of plant phenols, flavonoids and antioxidants with health benefits.

Put the rocket, endive, spring onions and kale in a mortar and roughly pound with the pestle, or process roughly in a processor.

Place the greens in a bowl. Add the fresh herbs and salted ricotta. Mix well to combine. Stir in the vinegar and season with salt and pepper.

Put the mixture on a serving plate and drizzle with the olive oil. Top with almonds and serve with olives and a slice of toasted sourdough bread.

VARIATIONS

In Ancient Rome, as well as adding a variety of chopped nuts to this dish, many other plants were eaten raw – watercress, mallow, sorrel, purslane, chicory, chervil, beetroot (beet) tops, celery tops, and many other herbs.

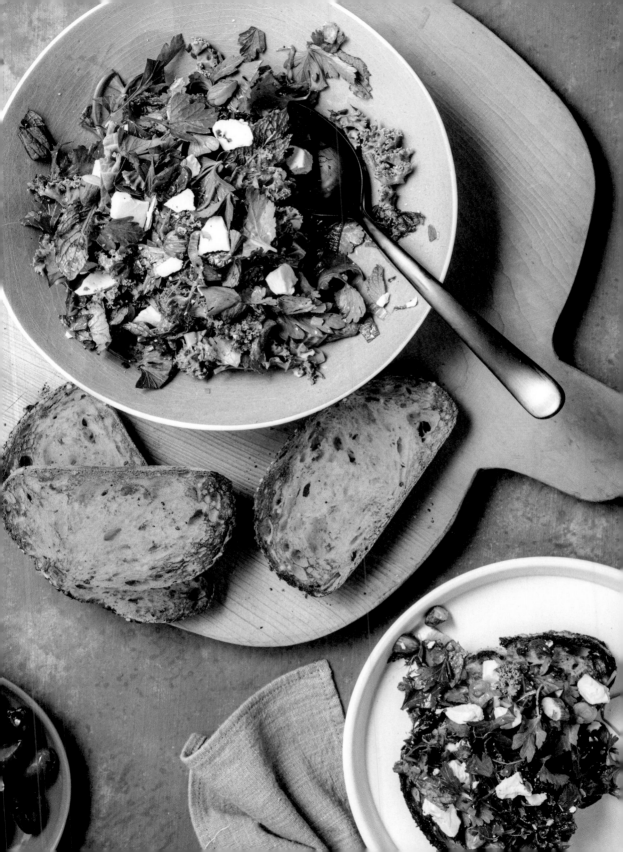

APPLE, AVOCADO AND ROCKET SALAD

2 apples, washed and cored, thinly sliced

2 large avocados, peeled, stone removed and sliced

70 g (2½ oz) baby rocket (arugula)

3 tablespoons freshly squeezed lemon juice

2 tablespoons extra-virgin olive oil

salt and freshly ground black pepper

2 large mint leaves, roughly torn

1 small hot chilli, seeds removed and finely chopped

A super-simple salad of two quite different fruits, one crunchy and sweet, the other creamy and soft.

Place the apple and avocado in a glass bowl and add the rocket. Season with lemon juice, olive oil and salt and pepper, and mix well. Garnish with the mint and chilli.

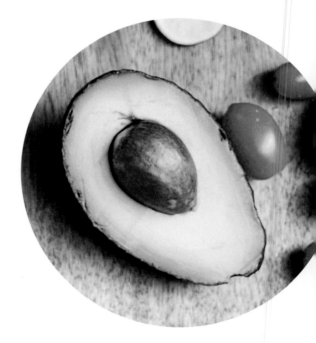

CAULIFLOWER AND OLIVE SALAD

SERVES **4** · PREPARATION TIME **15 MINUTES** · COOKING TIME **5–7 MINUTES**

600 g (1 lb 5 oz) cauliflower, cut into florets

100 g (3½ oz) black and green olives, pitted

1 teaspoon ground coriander

1 teaspoon ground turmeric

½ teaspoon ground ginger

80 ml (2½ fl oz/⅓ cup) extra-virgin olive oil

juice of ½ lemon

salt and freshly ground black pepper

Cauliflower, along with other cruciferous vegetables, provides antioxidants, phytonutrients and a number of anti-cancer compounds. These are vegetables you can also eat plenty of without worrying about putting on weight.

Bring a saucepan of salted water to the boil and boil the cauliflower until just tender. Drain and transfer to a bowl with the mixed olives. Add the spices and drizzle with the olive oil, lemon juice and season with salt and pepper. Toss to combine and serve.

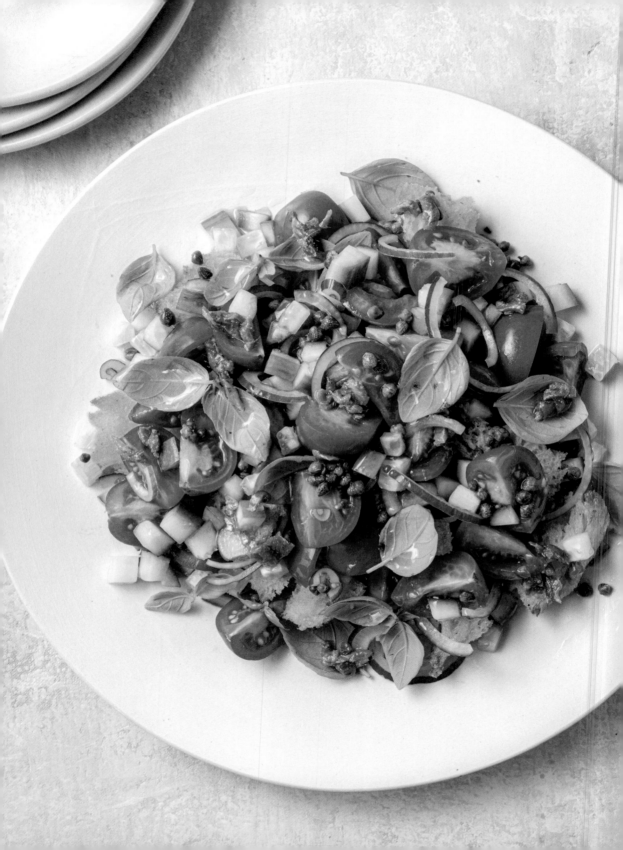

PANZANELLA
(TUSCAN TOMATO AND BREAD SALAD)

SERVES **4** • PREPARATION TIME **10 MINUTES**

4 slices stale wholemeal sourdough bread, crusts removed

300 g (10½ oz) ripe tomatoes, quartered or diced

1 small red onion, peeled and finely sliced

1 cucumber, diced

1 handful small capers, drained and rinsed

8 anchovy fillets in oil, drained and finely sliced

1 bunch basil

2 tablespoons extra-virgin olive oil

1 tablespoon white-wine vinegar

sea salt and freshly ground black pepper

Make this salad at least an hour before serving so the bread can absorb all the flavours. If the sourdough bread is fresh, tear it into pieces and place on a baking tray. Place in a 180°C (350°F) oven for 15 minutes to dry out.

Tear the bread into rough 2 cm (1 in) pieces and place in a salad bowl. Add the vegetables, capers, anchovies and basil leaves.

Drizzle with the olive oil and vinegar, and season with salt and pepper. Toss the mixture together with your hands. Cover and refrigerate for at least 1 hour before serving.

VARIATIONS

Add cos (romaine) lettuce leaves and radicchio leaves).

CABBAGE, WALNUT AND SULTANA SALAD

SERVES **4** · PREPARATION TIME **15 MINUTES**

400 g (14 oz) cabbage, finely chopped

100 g (3½ oz/1 cup) walnuts, finely chopped

2 tablespoons sultanas

80 ml (2½ fl oz/⅓ cup) extra-virgin olive oil

2 tablespoons apple-cider vinegar, or freshly squeezed lemon juice

salt and freshly ground black pepper

Cabbage contains antioxidants and phytochemicals (isothiocyanates) that have been shown to reduce chronic inflammation. And, surprisingly, cabbage is high in vitamin C and also both insoluble and soluble fibre, which help keep the gut healthy.

Combine the cabbage and walnuts in a bowl, then add the sultanas, olive oil, cider vinegar, salt and pepper. Toss to combine and serve.

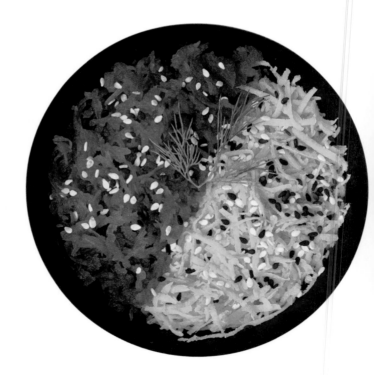

GRATED CARROT AND ORANGE SALAD

SERVES **4**
PREPARATION TIME **10 MINUTES**

4 large carrots, peeled and grated
juice of 3 oranges
3 tablespoons extra-virgin olive oil
2 teaspoons freshly ground cumin
salt and freshly ground black pepper
2 large mint leaves, finely shredded

As well as enriching food with its nutty flavour, freshly ground cumin also provides plenty of valuable polyphenols, among which the most prominent are quercetin, ellagic, syringic and p-coumaric acid. Very preliminary studies suggest some of these compounds might play a role in the prevention of cancer and diabetes.

Put the carrot in a bowl and add the orange juice, olive oil and cumin, and season to taste with salt and pepper. Toss to combine, then sprinkle with the mint leaves.

GRATED BEETROOT AND CARROT SALAD

SERVES **4**
PREPARATION TIME **15 MINUTES**

1 large carrot, peeled and grated
1 large beetroot (beet), peeled and grated
80 ml (2½ fl oz/⅓ cup) extra-virgin olive oil
2 tablespoons pomegranate juice, or orange juice
2 tablespoons apple-cider vinegar
salt and freshly ground black pepper
black and white sesame seeds, to serve

Colourful foods are a great way to ensure you are getting a range of different nutrients. Both carrots and beetroot are rich in beta carotene and a large number of other nutrients essential for good health.

Combine the carrot and beetroot in a bowl.

In another small bowl, whisk together the olive oil, pomegranate juice and cider vinegar. Pour over the carrot and beetroot, then season with salt and pepper. Toss to combine. Sprinkle with sesame seeds to serve.

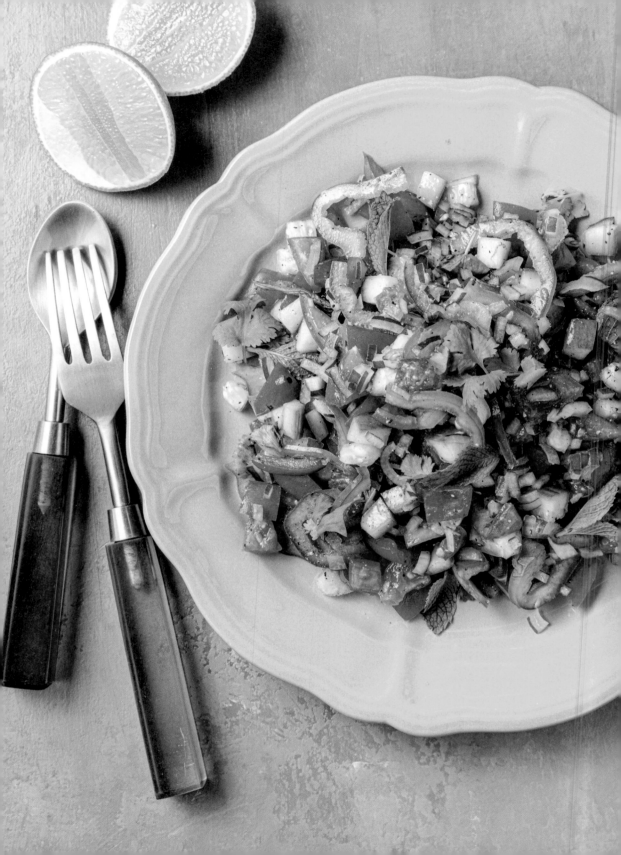

SHIRAZI SALAD

1 large cucumber,
  finely diced

3 ripe, firm tomatoes,
  deseeded and
  finely diced

¼ red onion, or
  3 spring onions
  (scallions),
  finely diced

2 tablespoons
  thinly sliced green
  capsicum (bell
  pepper), or mild
  green chilli pepper,
  deseeded

3 tablespoons roughly
  chopped coriander
  (cilantro), or parsley,
  dill or mint

3 tablespoons freshly
  squeezed lime juice

¼ teaspoon fine lime
  zest

2 tablespoons olive oil

salt and freshly
  ground black pepper

1 tablespoon chopped
  mint

A lot like the classic Mediterranean salad of tomato and cucumber, this Iranian salad is just a little more nuanced with green pepper and herbs.

Combine the cucumber, tomato and onion in a bowl. Add the pepper and coriander.

In a small cup, whisk together the lime juice and zest, olive oil, salt and pepper. Add the fresh mint. Drizzle over the salad ingredients and toss gently to combine.

WARM LENTIL AND ONION SALAD

SERVES **2** • PREPARATION TIME **10 MINUTES** • COOKING TIME **25 MINUTES**

185 g (6½ oz/1 cup) brown lentils

1 celery stick or celery leaves

pinch of salt

1 tablespoon extra-virgin olive oil

1 large onion, peeled and finely diced

1 garlic clove, peeled and finely chopped

½ teaspoon freshly ground cumin

½ teaspoon freshly ground coriander

⅓ teaspoon ground fenugreek

¼ teaspoon freshly ground cardamom

1 red chilli, thinly sliced

juice of ½ lemon

5 g (⅛ oz/¼ cup) finely chopped flat-leaf (Italian) parsley

Put the lentils in a pot with the celery and cover well with water. Bring to the boil, add a pinch of salt and cook gently until tender (see page 131). Drain the lentils, reserving 125 ml (4 fl oz/½ cup) cooking water. Discard the celery.

Heat the olive oil in a large saucepan over a low–medium heat and add the onion and garlic, spices and chilli. Sauté for 1–2 minutes, then add the lentils along with a couple of tablespoons of the cooking water. Cook for a few minutes until heated through, then add the lemon juice and parsley and mix well.

LENTIL, LEMON AND CHILLI SALAD

SERVES **4** • PREPARATION TIME **15 MINUTES** • COOKING TIME **25 MINUTES**

380 g (13½ oz) lentils

1 lemon, peeled and segmented

1 green chilli, seeds removed and finely sliced

80 ml (2½ fl oz/⅓ cup) extra-virgin olive oil

juice of ½ lemon

salt and freshly ground black pepper

Make these lentils as the basis for a salad bowl. Add any other salad ingredients including roasted vegetables, goat's cheese, grilled asparagus, Spicy chickpeas (see page 98), nuts and herbs – there are no end to combinations.

Put the lentils in a pot and cover well with water. Bring to the boil and cook gently until tender (see page 131). Drain and transfer to a bowl with the lemon and chilli. Add the olive oil and lemon juice, and season with salt and pepper. Toss to combine.

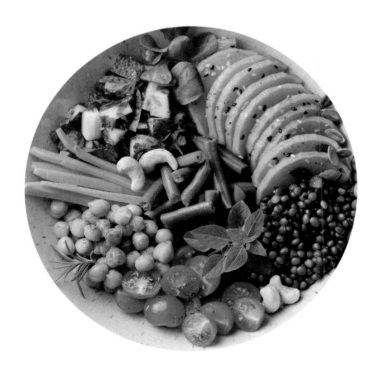

POMEGRANATE AND GREENS SALAD

SERVES **4** · PREPARATION TIME **10 MINUTES** · COOKING TIME **15 MINUTES**

100 g (3½ oz/½ cup) quinoa, rinsed

155 g (5½ oz/1 cup) peas

200 g (7 oz) asparagus, cut into 1 cm (½ in) pieces

200 g (7 oz) baby broccoli stems, cut into 1 cm (½ in) pieces

seeds of ½ pomegranate

2 tablespoons roughly torn basil leaves

2 tablespoons roughly chopped almonds

freshly ground black pepper

30 g (1 oz) goat's feta, crumbled

Pomegranate seeds get their vibrant red from polyphenols such as gallic acid, ellagic acid and punicalagin, which are powerful antioxidants.

Indeed, pomegranate juice contains three times the amount of potent antioxidants than green tea. These antioxidants help remove free radicals, protect cells from damage and reduce inflammation.

Bring 250 ml (8½ fl oz/1 cup) water to the boil in a saucepan. Add the quinoa, reduce to a simmer, cover with a lid and cook for 15 minutes, fluffing up the grains halfway through with a fork for extra volume. Cook until the grains are tender and the water has been absorbed. Set aside to cool.

Meanwhile, add the peas, asparagus and broccoli to a steamer set over a saucepan of simmering water and steam for 3–4 minutes, or until just tender. Set the vegetables aside.

Add the cooked quinoa, green vegetables and pomegranate seeds to a large bowl together with the basil and almonds, and mix well. Season with pepper. Sprinkle over the goat's feta.

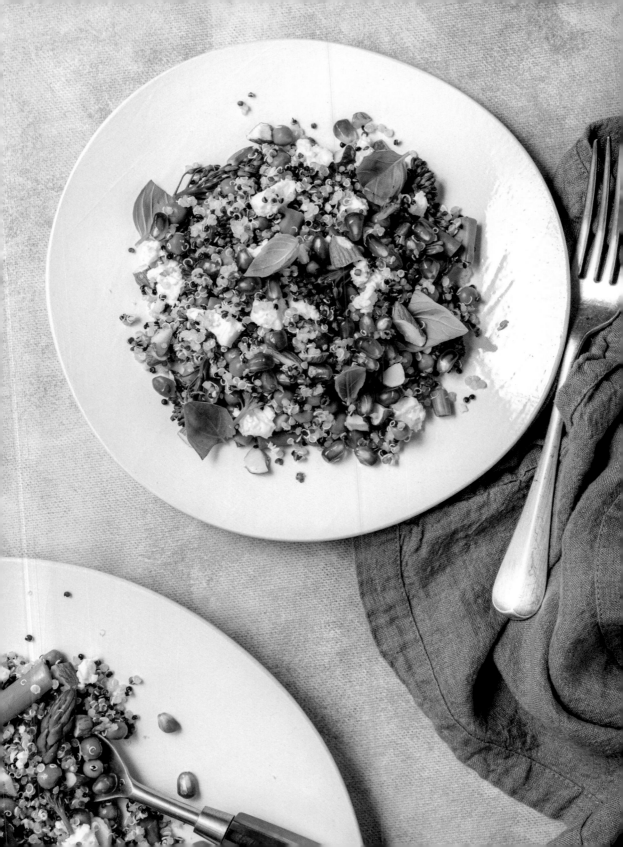

WARM SALAD OF BORLOTTI BEANS WITH GRILLED CARROTS AND ASPARAGUS

SERVES **4** · PREPARATION TIME **10 MINUTES** · COOKING TIME **15 MINUTES**

4 large carrots, peeled

12 asparagus spears, trimmed

1 tablespoon olive oil

1 teaspoon ground turmeric

salt and freshly ground black pepper

520 g (1 lb 2 oz/ 2 cups) cooked borlotti (cranberry) beans (see page 130–131)

head of red radicchio, finely sliced

10 cherry tomatoes, quartered

DRESSING

1 tablespoon extra-virgin olive oil

juice of ½ lemon

salt and freshly ground black pepper

Turmeric is one of my kitchen staples. It can be used fresh (grated) or dried and ground to give curries or vegetable dishes a distinctive sun-yellow colour and a slightly bitter, peppery, earthy taste. But, most importantly, this precious rhizome will provide high concentrations of a phytochemical called curcumin. Several studies show a potential anti-inflammatory, antioxidant and anti-cancer effect.

Preheat the oven to 190°C (375°F).

With a sharp knife, cut the carrots in half lengthways, and then cut each half lengthways again into two pieces. Place the carrots and asparagus in a baking dish and drizzle with olive oil. Sprinkle with the turmeric and season with salt and pepper. Bake in the oven for 15 minutes.

Meanwhile, combine the borlotti beans with the radicchio and cherry tomatoes in a salad bowl. Add the cooked carrots and asparagus, and dress with the olive oil, lemon juice and a pinch of salt and freshly ground black pepper.

HARICOT BEANS AND HARISSA SALAD

SERVES **4** · PREPARATION TIME **SOAKING OVERNIGHT, THEN 15 MINUTES**
COOKING TIME **40 MINUTES**

800 g (1 lb 12 oz) dried
  haricot beans

1 tablespoon harissa

4 tablespoons finely
  chopped flat-leaf
  (Italian) parsley

2 tablespoons olive oil

juice of ½ lemon

salt and freshly
  ground black pepper

Harissa is a Tunisian spice paste used around the Mediterranean. It can be added to many dishes, adding a spark of slightly sweet, smoky, spicy flavour.

Place the haricot beans in a bowl and cover with water. Leave to soak overnight. Drain, then place the haricot beans in a saucepan and cover with fresh water. Bring to the boil, then reduce to a gentle simmer and cook until tender, about 40 minutes. Drain and set aside.

Add the cooked haricot beans to a bowl with the harissa and parsley. Mix well to combine.

Add the oil and lemon juice, and season with salt and pepper.

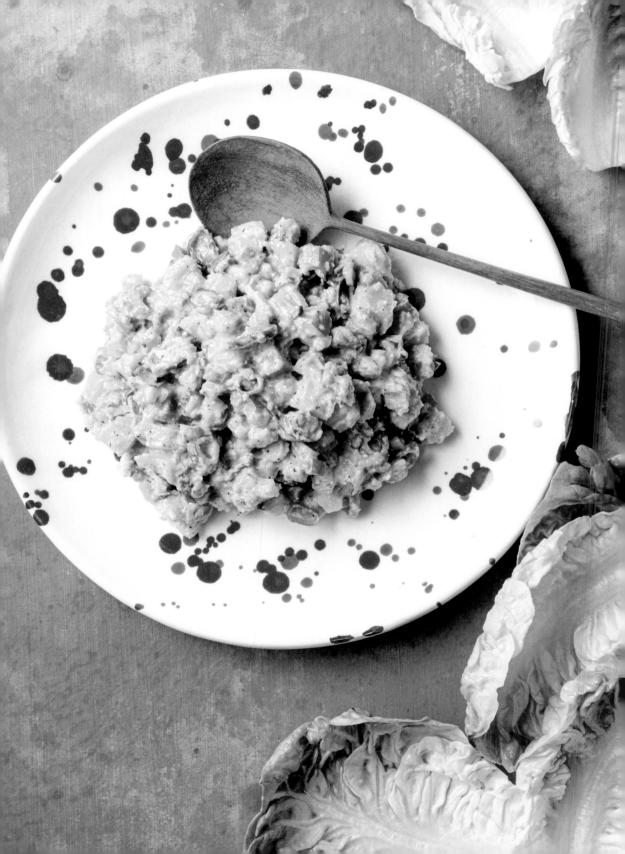

VEGAN SALAD

SERVES **4** • PREPARATION TIME **15 MINUTES**

8–10 carrots, peeled and roughly chopped

65 g (2¼ oz/¼ cup) tahini

1 teaspoon cumin seeds

pinch of salt

1 tablespoon extra-virgin olive oil

1 teaspoon lemon juice

3 spring onions (scallions), finely chopped

1 yellow or red capsicum (bell pepper), deseeded and diced

2 celery stalks, chopped

2 tablespoons finely chopped flat-leaf (Italian) parsley

lettuce, to serve

This creamy salad with chunks of onion, capsicum and celery is a little like a tuna mayonnaise salad but without the tuna or the mayo.

Place the carrots in a food processor and purée. Add the tahini, cumin, salt, the olive oil and lemon juice, and keep blending.

When the mixture is creamy, remove from the processor and add the chopped spring onions, capsicum, celery and parsley, and mix well. Taste and season accordingly. Serve with a lettuce salad or in lettuce cups.

SALAD BOWL OF MIXED GRAINS, CHICKPEAS AND GREEN BEANS

SERVES **2** · PREPARATION TIME **15 MINUTES** · COOKING TIME **35 MINUTES**

100 g (3½ oz) unpearled barley

50 g (1¾ oz/¼ cup) quinoa

1 tablespoon pine nuts

150 g (5½ oz) green beans

juice of ½ lemon, plus 1 tablespoon extra

3 tablespoons extra-virgin olive oil

6 basil leaves

65 g (2¼ oz) cooked chickpeas (see pages 130–131)

1 tablespoon tahini

1 bunch rocket (arugula)

4 cherry tomatoes

1 large avocado, peeled, stone removed and sliced

1 tablespoon sesame seeds

salt and freshly ground black pepper

Consuming legumes and unrefined grains has been shown to reduce glucose levels after a meal and also at subsequent meals. This effect is lost if we, instead, use highly milled grain flours or overcook legumes and grains at high temperatures. If we eat brown rice and lentils at lunch, our glycaemia at dinner will be lower. Or, even better, if we consume, for example, a quinoa and chickpea salad for dinner, our night-long blood glucose will be reduced. This subsequent-meal effect is very important not only for healthy individuals, but particularly for people with prediabetes and diabetes.

Pine nuts are an excellent source of vitamin E and contain high levels of arginine, an amino acid needed for the production of nitric oxide, which is essential for lowering blood pressure and preventing the aggregation of platelets.

Bring a saucepan of salted water to the boil. Add the barley and cook for 20 minutes, then add the quinoa and cook for a further 15 minutes, or until both the barley and quinoa are tender. Drain and transfer to a bowl.

Meanwhile, toast the pine nuts and in a dry frying pan over a medium heat. Be careful not to burn them. When done set aside.

Blanch the green beans in boiling water for a minute or two. Drain, and set aside in a small bowl to cool. Add 1 tablespoon lemon juice, 1 tablespoon of the olive oil, and the basil leaves.

In another small bowl, combine the cooked chickpeas with the tahini.

To serve, place the quinoa, barley and chickpeas in a salad bowl. Add the rocket, tomatoes, pine nuts, avocado and the green beans. Toss gently with your hands.

Dress with the remaining olive oil and lemon juice, sesame seeds and some salt and pepper.

BURGHUL TABOULEH SALAD

SERVES **4** • PREPARATION TIME **30 MINUTES**

300 g (10½ oz) burghul (bulgur wheat)

4 ripe tomatoes, finely chopped

4 small spring onions (scallions), finely chopped

1 bunch flat-leaf (Italian) parsley, finely chopped

1 tablespoon finely chopped mint

lettuce cups, to serve

DRESSING

2 tablespoons extra-virgin olive oil

3 tablespoons lemon juice

1 teaspoon sweet paprika

pinch of salt

Parsley is one of my favourite herbs. Because of its fresh, peppery and grassy flavour, it complements most other ingredients. Chopped parsley is the main ingredient in the Mediterranean salad tabouleh, and is essential in falafel. Parsley contains high levels of the flavone apigenin, which has been shown to inhibit the proliferation of tumour cells (at least in experiments conducted in cell culture systems). Other foods that are particularly rich in apigenin are onions, oranges, chamomile and wheat sprouts.

Place the burghul in a bowl and pour in enough hot water to cover it. Leave to stand for 30 minutes, or until softened. Drain and set aside.

For the dressing, in a bowl, mix together the olive oil, lemon juice, paprika and a pinch of salt. Add the burghul to the dressing to allow it to absorb some of the liquid.

Add the tomato, spring onion, parsley and mint to the burghul and mix well. Taste and adjust the seasoning as desired. Fill lettuce cups to serve.

VARIATIONS

This burghul mix can also be used to stuff baked vegetables, like capsicums (bell peppers) and zucchinis (courgettes). Top the stuffed vegetables with crumbled feta before baking.

BURGHUL WITH A PESTO OF HERBS AND NUTS

SERVES **4** • PREPARATION TIME **30 MINUTES**

300 g (10½ oz)
  burghul (bulgur
  wheat)

1 bunch basil

1 tablespoon chopped
  chives

1 tablespoon chopped
  mint

1 garlic clove, peeled

10 g (¼ oz) walnuts

2 tablespoons
  extra-virgin olive oil

2 tablespoons lemon
  juice

salt, to taste

6 almonds, finely
  chopped, to garnish

Walnuts are an excellent source of omega-3 alpha-linolenic acid, besides being a rich source of vitamin E and other polyphenols that may contribute to the prevention of oxidation of bad LDL-cholesterol particles. One hundred grams (3½ oz/1 cup) of walnuts provides two omega-3 fatty acids (also typical of healthy fish) that have cardio-protective properties, because they reduce inflammation and platelet aggregation.

Place the burghul in a bowl and pour in enough hot water to cover it. Leave to stand for 30 minutes, or until softened. Drain and set aside.

To make the pesto, put the basil, chives, mint, garlic, walnuts and olive oil in a food processor. Start blending and slowly add the lemon juice and enough water to achieve a creamy consistency. You might need to stop the blender occasionally to push the mixture down with a spatula.

Transfer the pesto to a large serving bowl and add the cooked burghul. Mix well, season with salt and top with the almonds.

MILLET SALAD

250 g (9 oz) millet

1 Lebanese cucumber, finely chopped

2 tomatoes, finely chopped

1 tablespoon chopped parsley

1 teaspoon chopped mint

2 tablespoons olive oil

juice of ½ lemon

salt and freshly ground black pepper

In a medium saucepan bring 250 ml (8 fl oz) water to the boil. Stir in the millet and reduce the heat to low. Cover and gently simmer for about 7 to 10 minutes until most of the water has been absorbed. Remove from the heat and let stand covered for about 10 minutes, until the millet is tender. With a fork fluff up the millet and transfer to a bowl.

Add the cucumber, tomato, parsley, mint, olive oil and lemon juice to the millet and toss. Season with salt and pepper and serve.

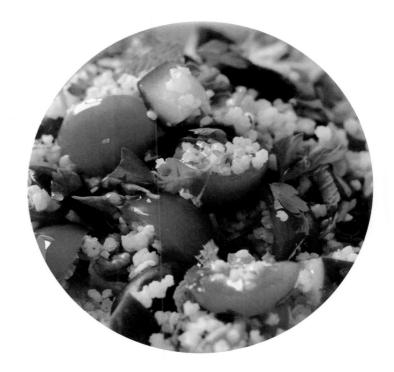

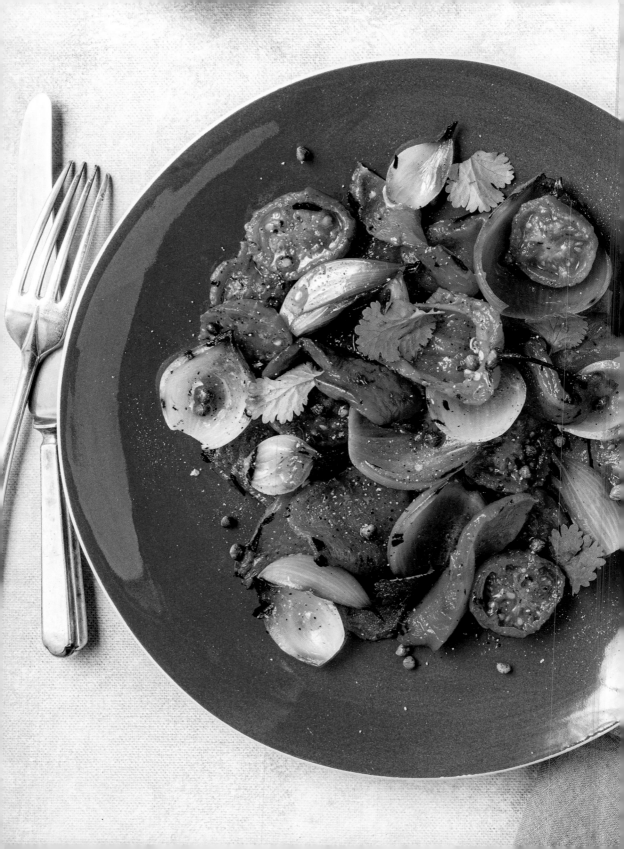

TUNISIAN GRILLED MECHOUIA SALAD

SERVES **6** · PREPARATION TIME **20 MINUTES** · COOKING TIME **25 MINUTES**

6 medium tomatoes, halved

4 red capsicums (bell peppers), halved and deseeded

1 large jalapeño chilli, halved and deseeded

3 small red onions, halved (skin on)

1 large garlic clove, crushed

2 tablespoons capers, chopped

1 teaspoon caraway seeds

½ teaspoon coriander seeds

3 tablespoons extra-virgin olive oil

juice of 1 lemon

salt and freshly ground black pepper

A simple dish from the Mediterranean of grilled vegetables is enhanced with Tunisian flavourings of chilli, spices and herbs.

Heat a chargrill pan or barbecue chargrill plate over a high heat and grill the tomatoes, capsicums, chilli and onions until the skin is blistered and blackened, about 10–20 minutes. Place the vegetables in a large bowl and cover with a plate to allow them to steam in their own heat for 15 minutes.

Peel the skins off the vegetables, reserving the juices left over in the bowl. Coarsely chop the vegetables and transfer to a serving bowl. Add the reserved juices, the garlic and capers.

Toast the caraway and coriander seeds in a small dry frying pan over a medium heat for a few minutes until they become fragrant. Grind them into a powder in a spice grinder or with a mortar and pestle. Combine the spices with the olive oil and lemon juice, then add to the chopped vegetables and stir well. Season to taste with salt and pepper.

VARIATIONS

You can garnish this dish with fresh parsley or coriander (cilantro), a hard-boiled egg, peeled and cut in quarters, half a cup of cooked tuna or a handful of olives.

FARRO, CUCUMBER AND RADISH SALAD

SERVES **4** • PREPARATION TIME **30 MINUTES** • COOKING TIME **40 MINUTES**

300 g (10½ oz/ 1½ cups) farro

750 ml (25½ fl oz/ 3 cups) vegetable broth

3 tablespoons extra-virgin olive oil

2 tablespoons fresh lemon juice

1 medium cucumber, peeled and diced

6 spring onions (scallions), sliced

6 radishes, trimmed and sliced

2 tablespoons finely chopped red onion

1 tablespoon chopped basil

1 tablespoon chopped flat-leaf (Italian) parsley

pinch of Aleppo pepper

pinch of chilli flakes

salt and freshly ground black pepper

Farro is an ancient wheat grain that originated in Mesopotamia thousands of years ago. It's packed with fibre, protein, vitamins, selenium and powerful antioxidants such as ferulic acid. Farro is particularly popular in Italy.

Place the farro in a glass bowl and cover with cool water. Soak for 60 minutes. Drain the farro and transfer to a saucepan with the vegetable broth. Bring to the boil. Skim any foam that rises to the surface with a spoon, then reduce the heat to very low, add a pinch of salt, cover, and simmer until the farro kernels become tender, about 30–40 minutes.

Drain and transfer the farro to a salad bowl and, immediately, while the farro is still hot, dress with 2 tablespoons of the olive oil and 1 tablespoon of the lemon juice. Set aside for 30 minutes to let the wheat absorb all the flavours.

Add all the remaining ingredients and mix well. Before serving, dress with the remaining olive oil and lemon juice, and season with salt and pepper.

BARLEY, CHICKPEA AND ROCKET SALAD

SERVES **4–6** • PREPARATION TIME **SOAKING 60 MINUTES, THEN 20 MINUTES**
COOKING TIME **40 MINUTES**

330 g (11½ oz/1½ cups)
  unpearled barley

750 ml (25½ fl oz/
  3 cups) vegetable
  stock

pinch of salt

225 g (8 oz/5 cups)
  rocket (arugula)

170 g (6 oz/1 cup)
  cooked chickpeas
  (see pages 130–131)

1 large cucumber,
  peeled and diced

2 red capsicums
  (bell peppers),
  cored and chopped

20 kalamata olives,
  pitted and sliced
  into thin rounds

2 tablespoons finely
  chopped red onion

15 g (½ oz/½ cup)
  chopped flat-leaf
  (Italian) parsley

75 g (2¾ oz/½ cup)
  crumbled feta

DRESSING

3 tablespoons
  extra-virgin olive oil

2 tablespoons fresh
  lemon juice

2 garlic cloves, crushed

pinch of dried
  oregano

pinch of chilli flakes

salt and freshly
  ground black pepper

One way to increase iron and zinc absorption is to add vitamin C. It is always a good idea to use lemon juice to dress and season vegetables, legumes and grains, because it helps to increase the absorption of many minerals and oligoelements. Just a generous squeeze of lemon juice improves how our gut absorbs iron and calcium from plant sources. The saying 'always add lemon' is a good mantra to live by.

Place the barley in a glass bowl and cover with cool water. Soak for 60 minutes. Drain the barley and transfer to a saucepan with the vegetable stock. Bring to the boil. Skim any foam that rises to the surface, then reduce the heat to a low simmer. Add a pinch of salt, cover, and simmer until the barley kernels become tender, about 30–40 minutes. Top up the water if needed.

Meanwhile, in a separate small bowl, combine the dressing ingredients and season to taste with salt and pepper.

Once cooked, drain the barley and transfer to a bowl. While the barley is hot, add the dressing so it absorbs the flavours. Toss and set aside to cool.

In a large serving bowl, combine the rocket, chickpeas, cucumber, capsicum, olives, onion and parsley. Add the cooled barley to the salad. Mix well and add the feta, then toss again and season to taste with more salt and pepper, if needed.

VARIATIONS

Instead of feta you could use buffalo mozzarella.

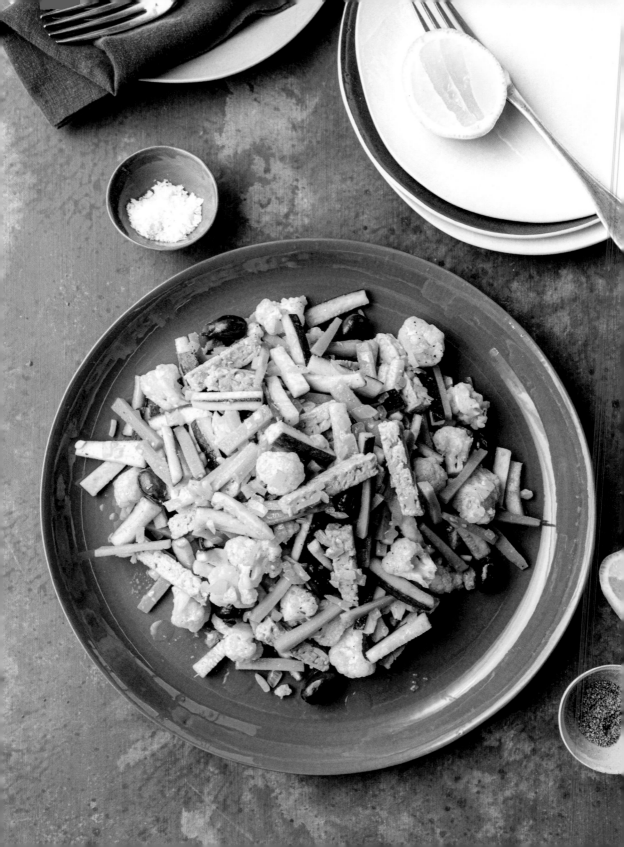

RAINBOW TEMPEH SALAD

SERVES **4** • PREPARATION TIME **20 MINUTES** • COOKING TIME **30 MINUTES**

½ cauliflower head

2 tablespoons
extra-virgin olive oil

1 small onion, finely
diced

1 teaspoon ground
turmeric

2 carrots, cut into thin
batons

2 zucchinis
(courgettes), cut
into thin batons

200 g (7 oz) tempeh,
cut into thin batons

50 g (1¾ oz) olives,
pitted

2 tablespoons fresh
lemon juice

salt and freshly
ground black pepper

Tempeh is made from fermented soybeans. It is high in protein and offers a host of different vitamins and minerals, like calcium, manganese, phosphorus and iron.

Cut the cauliflower into small florets and place in a steamer. Steam until just cooked, then set aside.

In a large non-stick frying pan heat the olive oil over a medium heat. Add the onion and turmeric and sauté for 1 minute, then add the finely sliced carrots and zucchini. Sauté for a few minutes until softening, then add the tempeh and cauliflower and toss through. Lastly, add the olives and lemon juice and cook for another 10 minutes. Season to taste, then serve.

PASTA

CLAM SPAGHETTI

SERVES **4** • PREPARATION TIME **SOAKING 2–3 HOURS, THEN 10 MINUTES**
COOKING TIME **15 MINUTES**

1 kg (2 lb 3 oz) small clams, from a sustainable source

salt, for soaking

400 g (14 oz) dried spaghetti

2 tablespoons extra-virgin olive oil, plus extra for drizzling

4 garlic cloves, finely chopped

freshly ground black pepper

1–2 dried red chillies

10 cherry tomatoes, chopped

½ bunch flat-leaf (Italian) parsley, finely chopped

Shellfish are a great source of lean protein, healthy fats (omega-3) and minerals like iron, zinc, magnesium and vitamin B12 (that is extremely important for the prevention of anemia).

Rinse the clams in cold running water. Put them into a large bowl and cover with cold water. Salt generously and leave for 2–3 hours, then drain and rinse well to remove any grit or sand. Sort through your cleaned clams and if there are any that aren't tightly closed, give them a sharp tap. If they don't close, throw them away.

In the meantime, heat a large saucepan of water for the pasta. Once boiling, add the pasta with a good pinch of salt and cook according to the packet instructions until al dente (usually about 10 minutes).

Heat a shallow, heavy-bottomed pan (that has a lid) over a high heat with the olive oil. Add the garlic and a good pinch of salt and pepper. Crumble in the dried chilli and add the cherry tomato. Stir, and as soon as the garlic starts to colour, add the clams. It will splutter and steam, so give everything a good shake, and put the lid on the pan. After about 3–4 minutes the clams will start to open, so keep moving them around in the pan until they have all opened. Take the pan off the heat. Remove any clams that haven't opened. This should all only take a few minutes.

Drain the pasta and add to the clams along with the finely chopped parsley and an extra drizzle of olive oil. Toss the clams through the pasta to allow the flavours to be absorbed for a minute or two. Serve immediately.

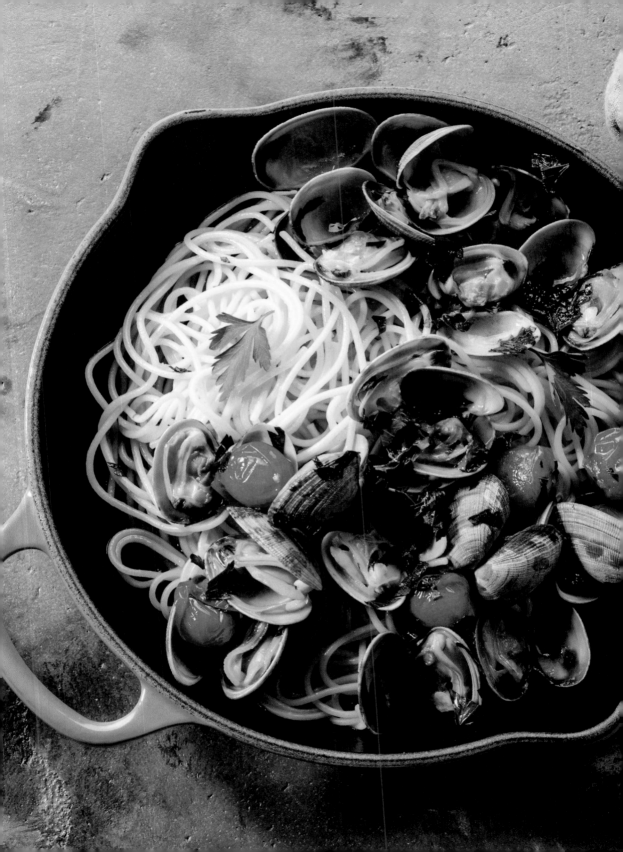

SPAGHETTI WITH A SIMPLE FRESH TOMATO SAUCE

SERVES **4** · PREPARATION TIME **10 MINUTES** · COOKING TIME **10 MINUTES**

200 g (7 oz/1 cup) chopped ripe tomatoes

2 garlic cloves, finely chopped

50 g (1¾ oz) flat-leaf (Italian) parsley, finely chopped

80 ml (2½ fl oz/⅓ cup) extra-virgin olive oil

salt, to taste

320 g (11½ oz) dried spaghetti

grated parmesan, to serve (optional)

There are two basic varieties of wheat: 'hard', or durum, and 'soft', plus other subspecies, such as spelt or farro – one of the oldest cereal grains.

Durum wheat has more protein than soft wheat and is used to make pasta. It contains high levels of an elastic protein called gluten and is a nutritious cereal that has been eaten in Mediterranean diets for centuries. For modern diets, a maximum of 100 g (3½ oz) pasta per serve is ideal. Whole-wheat or wholemeal spaghetti has a lower glycaemic index.

There are other ways to make good use of this nutritious cereal. It can be eaten as couscous, a staple food of many regions facing the Mediterranean Sea, especially in North Africa and Sicily. Couscous is made from semolina, the coarse grind of high-protein durum wheat. Whole-wheat couscous is more nutritious than the regular variety.

In a large bowl, mix together the tomato, garlic and parsley. Add the olive oil and some salt, and mix well. Let stand at room temperature so that the oil soaks into the ingredients.

In the meantime, heat a large saucepan of water for the pasta. Once boiling, add the pasta with a good pinch of salt and cook according to the packet instructions until al dente (usually about 10 minutes).

Drain the pasta and add to the tomato and garlic sauce. Mix well and serve with grated parmesan, if using.

PENNE WITH
FRESH TOMATO, OLIVE AND CAPER SAUCE

SERVES **4** • PREPARATION TIME **10 MINUTES** • COOKING TIME **10 MINUTES**

200 g (7 oz/1 cup) chopped ripe cherry tomatoes

95 g (3¼ oz) chopped black olives

110 g (4 oz/½ cup) chopped green olives

20 g (¾ oz) capers, chopped

2 garlic cloves, finely chopped

15 g (½ oz) flat-leaf (Italian) parsley, finely chopped

80 ml (2½ fl oz/⅓ cup) extra-virgin olive oil

salt, to taste

320 g (11½ oz) dried penne pasta

grated parmesan, to serve (optional)

Capers are grown around the Mediterranean, particularly in Italy, Malta and Greece, and have many health benefits, some of which we are only just learning about. They are rich in quercetin and vitamin K and have been linked to bone health and decreased levels of cholesterol. They have also been shown to fight free radicals, aiding the prevention of chronic disease.

Mix together the tomatoes, olives, capers, garlic and parsley in a large bowl and add the olive oil and salt. Let stand at room temperature so that the oil soaks into the ingredients.

In the meantime, heat a large saucepan of water for the pasta. Once boiling, add the pasta with a good pinch of salt and cook according to the packet instructions until al dente (usually about 10 minutes). Drain and add to the bowl of ingredients. Mix well and serve right away with grated parmesan, if using.

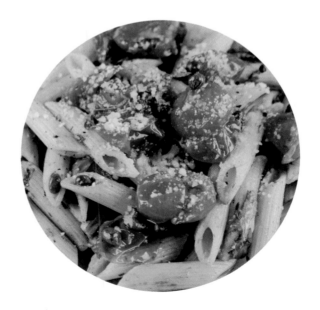

SPAGHETTI WITH TRAPANESE PESTO

SERVES **4** • PREPARATION TIME **15 MINUTES** • COOKING TIME **10 MINUTES**

50 g (1¾ oz/⅓ cup) almonds, peeled

250 g (9 oz) ripe tomatoes, deseeded and chopped

50 g (1¾ oz) basil leaves

1 garlic clove, finely chopped

100 ml (3½ fl oz) extra-virgin olive oil, plus extra for drizzling

320 g (11½ oz) dried spaghetti

salt, to taste

grated pecorino, to serve

This is more like a sauce than a pesto, but the almonds add to the texture.

Put the almonds in a small bowl and cover with boiling water. Set aside for 5 minutes, then drain them. Squeeze the wrinkly skin off the almonds between your fingers and the peel should easily come off.

Put the almonds, chopped tomato, basil, garlic and oil in a food processor and blend.

Transfer the pesto to a serving bowl, reserving 2 tablespoons.

Fill a large saucepan with water and bring to the boil. Add the spaghetti with a good pinch of salt and cook according to the packet instructions until al dente (usually about 10 minutes).

Drain the pasta and pour over the pesto in the serving bowl. Add a drizzle of extra-virgin olive oil and top with a small amount of grated pecorino. Mix everything well and serve with the remaining pesto on top.

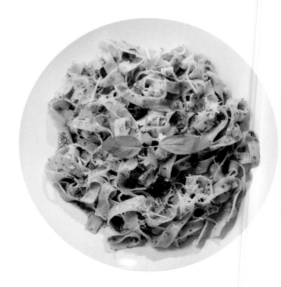

TAGLIATELLE WITH SIMPLE PESTO

SERVES **4** · PREPARATION TIME **20 MINUTES** · COOKING TIME **10 MINUTES**

320 g (11½ oz) dried tagliatelle

SIMPLE PESTO

2 garlic cloves, finely chopped

2 pinches coarse salt

50 g (1¾ oz) basil leaves

15 g (½ oz) pine nuts

70 g (2½ oz) grated parmesan

100 ml (3½ fl oz) extra-virgin olive oil

For a flavour hit, pesto can be drizzled over almost any savoury dish, stirred into soups, mixed with cooked beans or chickpeas.

To make the pesto, crush the garlic with a mortar and pestle together with a few grains of coarse salt until it becomes a cream. Add the basil leaves along with another pinch of coarse salt – which will serve to crush the fibres better and maintain a nice bright-green colour – and pound until a bright-green paste develops. Add the pine nuts and crush them into the paste until you obtain a cream. Add the grated cheese, a little at a time, stirring continuously. Finally, add the olive oil, stirring with the pestle until it is all well blended. Work through this process quite quickly to avoid oxidation.

If you do not have a mortar and pestle or prefer to use a food processor, it is best to use the plastic blades, because the metal blades do not release all the flavour from the leaves and can result in a bitter pesto. And it is also better to run the blender at the lowest speed and use the pulse function to avoid heating the leaves and discolouring the pesto. Another precaution to avoid the pesto overheating is to put the blender cup and blades in the refrigerator 1 hour before use.

For the pasta, bring a large saucepan of water to the boil. Add the pasta with a good pinch of salt and cook according to the packet instructions until al dente (usually about 10 minutes).

Drain, then transfer the pasta to a bowl and fold through the pesto sauce. Serve immediately.

NOTE

The basil leaves need to be dry (dry with a soft cloth) and must not be damaged as this can cause oxidation, making the pesto dark green with a herbaceous aroma.

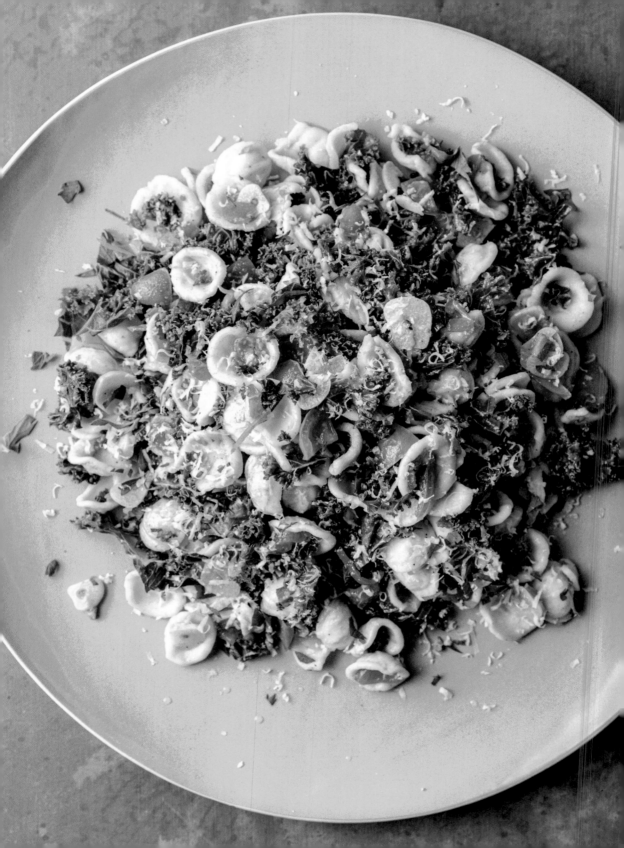

ORECCHIETTE WITH RAPINI OR KALE

SERVES **4** · PREPARATION TIME **10 MINUTES** · COOKING TIME **10 MINUTES**

250 g (9 oz)
  orecchiette

2 pinches of salt

2 tablespoons
  extra-virgin olive
  oil, plus extra for
  drizzling

3 garlic cloves, sliced

freshly ground black
  pepper

½ red chilli, sliced

10 cherry tomatoes,
  chopped

5 anchovies

200 g (7 oz) rapini or
  kale, coarsely sliced

1 tablespoon finely
  chopped flat-leaf
  (Italian) parsley

grated parmesan,
  to serve (optional)

Dark leafy greens are considered great sources of healthy antioxidants, folic acid, vitamins and fibre. Rapini is a favourite in the Mediterranean.

Fill a large saucepan with water and bring to the boil. Add the orecchiette with a good pinch of salt and cook according to the packet instructions until al dente (usually about 10 minutes).

In the meantime, heat the olive oil in non-stick frying pan over a medium heat and add the garlic and a good pinch of salt and pepper. Add the chilli and the chopped tomatoes. Stir well and, just as the garlic starts to colour, add the anchovies and stir to combine. Set aside.

Two minutes before the pasta is ready, add the rapini to the pasta to cook. Once cooked, drain the pasta and rapini, then add it to the sauce and toss to coat over a high heat. Garnish with the parsley and an extra drizzle of olive oil. Serve with grated parmesan, if using.

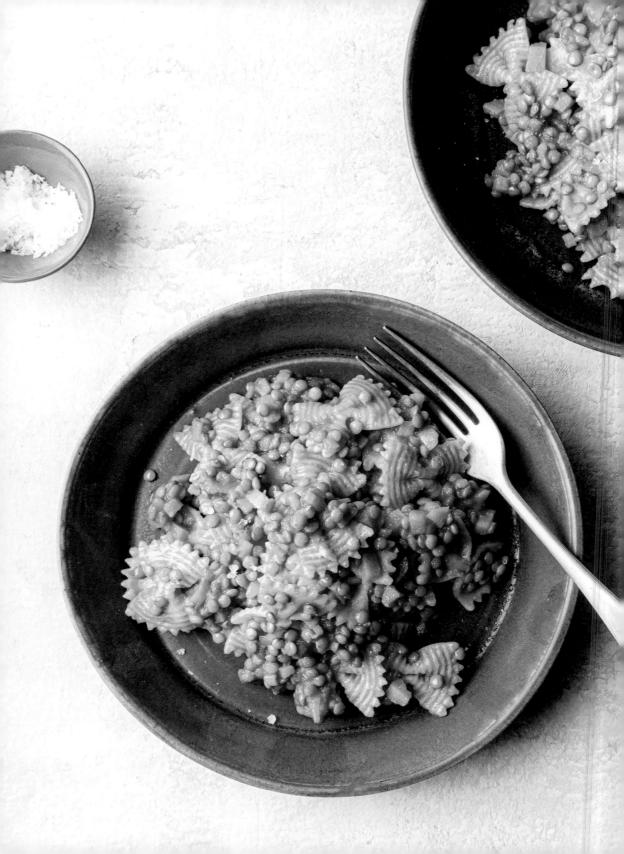

FARFALLE PASTA WITH LENTIL RAGOUT

SERVES **4** · PREPARATION TIME **20 MINUTES** · COOKING TIME **30 MINUTES**

80 ml (2½ fl oz/⅓ cup) extra-virgin olive oil

1 garlic clove, finely chopped

2 tablespoons finely chopped celery

½ onion, finely chopped

pinch of chilli powder

2 pinches of salt

2 carrots, chopped

2 tablespoons freshly squeezed lemon juice

300 g (10½ oz) red lentils, rinsed

700 g (1 lb 9 oz) tomato passata (puréed tomatoes)

320 g (11½ oz) farfalle pasta

freshly ground black pepper

A combination of legumes and whole grains provides all the essential amino acids needed to form healthy proteins in our body, without the saturated fatty acids that promote plaque in our arteries. Unlike animal products and vegetable oils, they do not contain any saturated or trans-fatty acids, or other unhealthy ingredients.

A meal of brown rice and chickpeas, or durum wheat pasta with lentils provides a complete protein – no different from the protein found in eggs or meat.

Heat the olive oil in a non-stick frying pan over a medium heat and add the garlic, celery, onion, chilli powder and a pinch of salt. Stir for 1 minute. Add the chopped carrots and lemon juice and keep stirring until the carrots soften.

Add the lentils (they do not need to be soaked), the passata and 750 ml (25½ fl oz/3 cups) water. Stir and raise the heat slightly, then cook for about 20 minutes or until the lentils are tender.

Fill a large saucepan with water and bring it to the boil. Add the farfalle to the boiling water with a good pinch of salt and cook according to packet instructions until al dente (usually about 10 minutes).

Drain the pasta, reserving a little of the cooking water, then add to the pan with the lentils and mix well. If it's a little dry, add some of the reserved cooking water. Serve immediately.

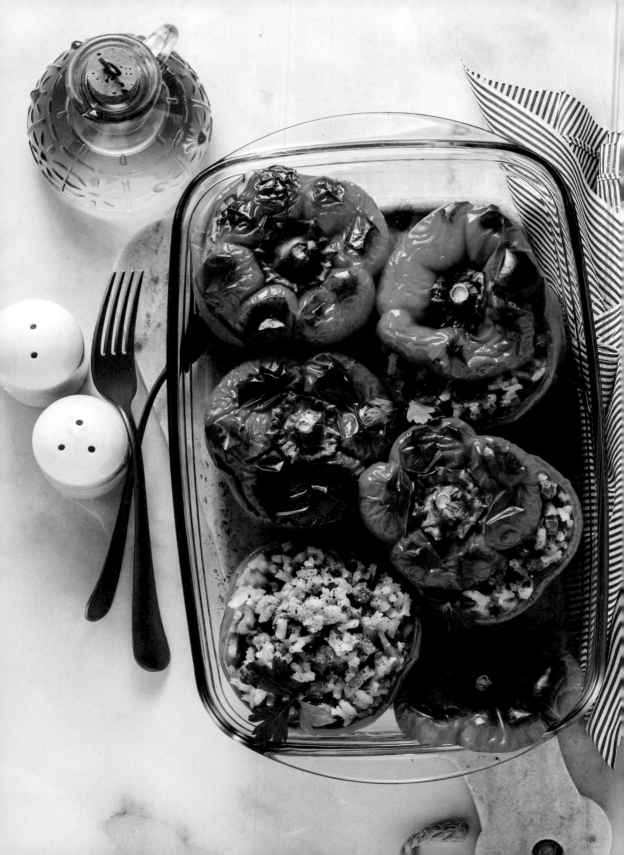

PLANT-BASED DISHES AND SIDES

ALMOND AND BROWN RICE-STUFFED PEPPERS

SERVES **4** · PREPARATION TIME **15 MINUTES** · COOKING TIME **1 HOUR 10 MINUTES**

95 g (3⅓ oz) brown rice

4 small to medium red or yellow capsicums (bell peppers)

2 tablespoons extra-virgin olive oil

1 small carrot, peeled and finely diced

2 garlic cloves, finely chopped

1 small shallot, finely chopped

½ teaspoon dried chilli

2 tablespoons peas

2 tablespoons finely chopped flat-leaf (Italian) parsley

75 g (2¾ oz) almonds, finely chopped

1 tablespoon capers, finely chopped

½ teaspoon salt

50 g (1¾ oz/⅓ cup) crumbled feta cheese or diced mozzarella cheese (optional)

Brown rice is highly nutritious and high in magnesium and selenium, and also contains a wide array of vitamins and oligoelements as well as antioxidants. Many vegetables can be stuffed: eggplants (aubergines), zucchini (courgettes), even sweet potatoes can be lightly roasted and then stuffed, and returned to the oven to bake until done.

Place the rice in a saucepan with 750 ml (25½ fl oz/3 cups) water. Heat to a simmer then cook for 45 minutes or until tender. Drain and set aside to cool.

Preheat the oven to 180°C (350°F).

Remove the tops of the capsicums and scoop out the seeds and veins. Place capsicums, with their tops on, in a baking dish and bake until just softened, about 15 minutes. Remove and set aside.

Heat 1 tablespoon of the olive oil in a small saucepan. Add the carrot and saute for 2–3 minutes, then add the garlic, shallot, and chilli and sauté for another minute. Stir in the peas and chopped parsley and remove from the heat.

In a small bowl, combine the brown rice, almonds, capers and salt with the garlic mixture. Stir in 1 tablespoon of the olive oil.

Gently fill the peppers with the stuffing and place the filled peppers on a baking tray. Sprinkle with feta or mozzarella, if using, and place tops on the capsicums. Bake uncovered for 20–25 minutes.

VEGETARIAN BOLOGNESE

SERVES **4** • PREPARATION TIME **20 MINUTES** • COOKING TIME **50 MINUTES**

1 tablespoon olive oil

2 carrots, finely chopped

1 onion, finely chopped

2 garlic cloves, finely chopped

500 g (1 lb 2 oz) Swiss brown mushrooms, finely chopped

400 g (14 oz) brown lentils, cooked

400 g (14 oz) whole tomatoes

grated parmesan, to serve (optional)

finely chopped flat-leaf (Italian) parsley, to serve

Eating plenty of nutrient-rich vegetables daily and subsequently feeling full means that you simply have less room for food you don't need. This is a hearty warming Bolognese-style stew that can be served on its own, over pasta, or with other vegetables.

Heat a heavy-bottomed saucepan over a medium heat. Add the olive oil and sauté the carrot, onion and garlic until soft. Stir in the mushrooms and cook for 10 minutes, stirring regularly.

Add the cooked lentils and the tomatoes with 400 ml (13½ fl oz) water. Bring to a simmer, cover with a lid and cook slowly for 40 minutes.

This can be served on its own with a salad or over pasta. Serve with a sprinkle of parmesan cheese, if desired, and finely chopped parsley.

POLENTA SLICES WITH PESTO

SERVES **4** · PREPARATION TIME **10 MINUTES** · COOKING TIME **50 MINUTES**

750 ml (25½ oz/3 cups)
vegetable stock
(optional)

150 g (5½ oz/1 cup)
polenta (not quick-
cooking)

½ teaspoon salt

1 tablespoon
extra-virgin olive oil,
plus extra for oiling

Simple pesto (page
85)

4 tomatoes, diced

1 bunch basil

Polenta is a delicious and versatile traditional northern Italian cornmeal dish that can be topped with any pasta sauce, sautéed greens or mushrooms, tomatoes or a lentil or bean stew. It's also great for breakfast.

Combine 750 ml (25½ fl oz/3 cups) cold water or vegetable stock if using, the polenta and salt in a saucepan and bring to the boil over a high heat. Once it starts to bubble, whisk the polenta frequently so it doesn't become lumpy. Reduce the heat to low–medium and cook, stirring constantly with a long-handled wooden spoon, until the polenta begins to pull away from the side of pan, roughly 30–45 minutes.

Pour the polenta into a pre-oiled glass dish, smoothing out the top in an even layer. Let it cool, then cover and place in the refrigerator for at least 3 hours, or overnight.

Remove the polenta from the fridge and slice it into squares or rectangles. Lightly oil the polenta, then in a chargrill pan or on a barbecue chargrill plate over a high heat, cook until golden brown, about 3 minutes on each side.

Top the grilled polenta slices with a drizzle of pesto and sprinkle with diced tomatoes, basil leaves and a drizzle of olive oil.

ROASTED VEGETABLES AND COUSCOUS

SERVES **4** • PREPARATION TIME **30 MINUTES** • COOKING TIME **30 MINUTES**

1 tablespoon olive oil, plus extra for drizzling

¼ butternut pumpkin (squash), peeled, deseeded and cut into 2 cm (¾ in) pieces

½ eggplant (aubergine), cut into 2 cm (¾ in) cubes

1 zucchini (courgette), cut into 2 cm (¾ in) pieces

140 g (5 oz/¾ cup) couscous

½ red onion, finely sliced

½ red capsicum (bell pepper), roughly diced

150 g (5½ oz/3⅓ cups) baby rocket (arugula)

squeeze of lemon juice

salt and freshly ground black pepper

Vegetables of all kinds can be tray-baked in a little olive oil. Vegetables can include parsnips, carrots, onions, asparagus, sweet potato, broccoli, cauliflower, eggplant (aubergine), zucchini (courgette) and many more. Sprinkled with herbs like thyme and rosemary and ground black pepper or dried chilli, with garlic cloves scattered among the veggies, it is a delicious and warming dish that can be eaten on its own or mixed with a grain such as couscous.

Preheat the oven to 200°C (400°F). Pour the olive oil in the bottom of a deep baking tray. Add the pumpkin pieces and toss. Bake for 10 minutes, then add the eggplant and zucchini, so all the vegetables are in a single layer, and roast for a further 20 minutes, or until cooked. Remove from the oven and set aside.

Meanwhile, combine the couscous and 185 ml (6 fl oz) boiling water in a bowl, mix with a fork, cover with a plate and leave to stand for 7 minutes. When the vegetables are done, fluff the couscous with a fork. Mix together the roasted vegetables, onion, capsicum, couscous and rocket. Dress with a drizzle of olive oil and a squeeze of lemon juice. Season to taste.

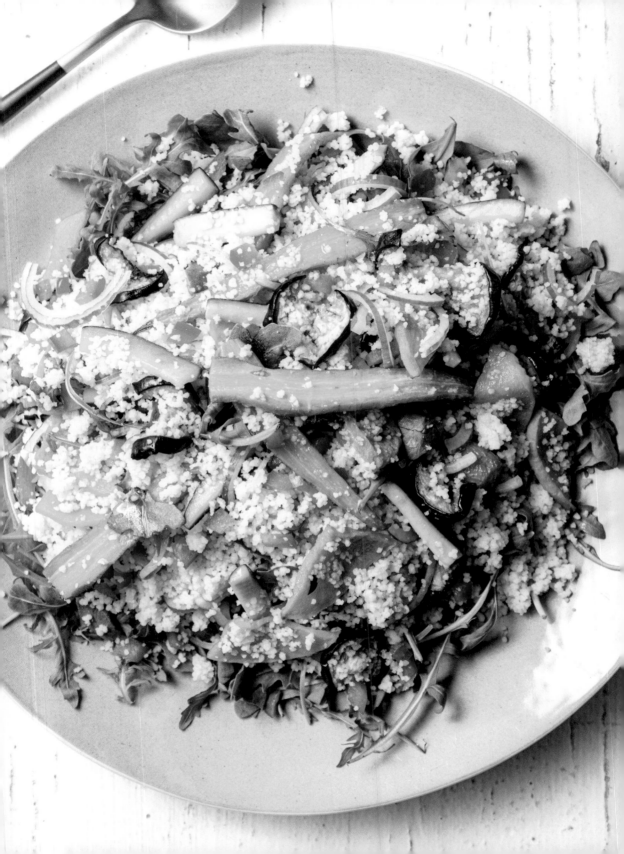

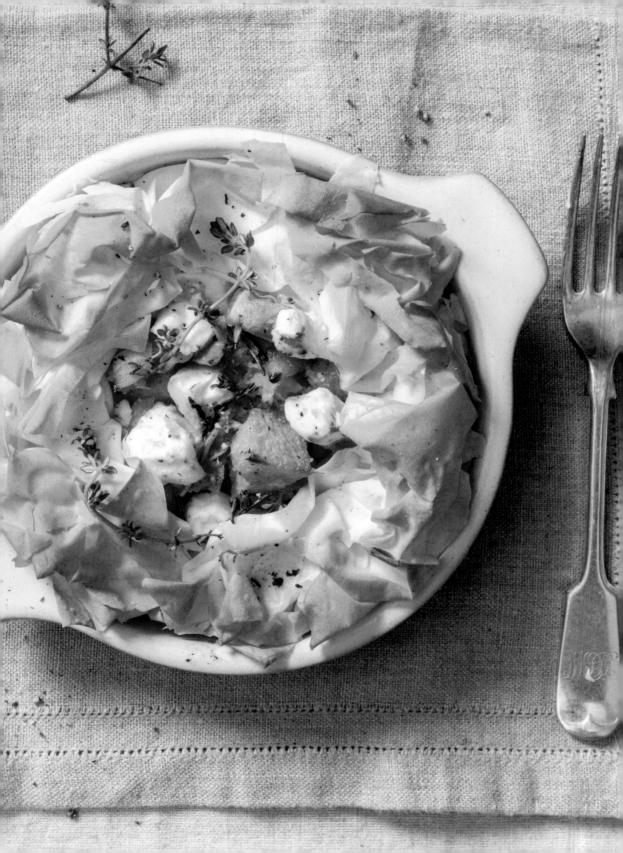

BAKED PUMPKIN AND FETA FILO PIE

SERVES **4** • PREPARATION TIME **10 MINUTES** • COOKING TIME **1 HOUR 10 MINUTES**

500 g (1 lb 2 oz) butternut pumpkin (squash), peel removed

2 tablespoons olive oil

1 onion, finely chopped

3 sprigs rosemary, finely chopped

4 free-range eggs

8 sheets filo pastry

salt and freshly ground black pepper

120 g (4½ oz) feta cheese, or diced mozzarella cheese

You can also make this pie with greens, by replacing the pumpkin (winter squash) with a bunch of spinach or kale that has been lightly steamed.

Preheat the oven to 180°C (350°F).

Coarsely chop the pumpkin into chunks of about 2.5 cm (1 inch) and place in a baking dish. Bake for about 30 minutes until the pumpkin is cooked. Set aside to cool. Leave the oven on.

In the meantime, heat a frying pan over a medium heat, add 1 tablespoon of the olive oil and sauté the onion until softened and beginning to brown. Remove from the heat and pour into a large bowl to cool. When cool, add the rosemary and mix in the cooled pumpkin.

In another bowl, beat the eggs well. Season with salt and pepper.

Layer the filo in a 23 cm (9 in) round pie dish, basting lightly with the remaining olive oil. Leave some of each sheet of filo hanging over the edge of the pie dish by about 10 cm (4 in). (This will be folded back over the pie when the dish is filled.) Add the cooled vegetables to the filo-lined pie dish. Pour over the egg and crumble over the feta or mozzarella cheese. Fold the edges of the filo over the pie. It doesn't need to cover the dish.

Bake for 40 minutes until nicely browned and the middle has set.

Serve slices with a green salad.

SPICY CHICKPEAS
WITH TOMATOES AND SPINACH

SERVES **4** • PREPARATION TIME **10 MINUTES** • COOKING TIME **25 MINUTES**

600 g (1 lb 5 oz) spinach

2 tablespoons extra-virgin olive oil

1 onion, peeled and finely chopped

3 garlic cloves, finely chopped

2 tablespoons ground turmeric

2 teaspoons ground coriander

2 teaspoons ground cumin

½ teaspoon finely chopped red chilli

2 tablespoons tomato paste (concentrated purée)

400 g (14 oz) tomatoes, chopped

300 g (10½ oz) cooked chickpeas (see pages 130–131)

salt, to taste

1 tablespoon low-fat Greek-style yoghurt

1 teaspoon finely chopped mint

Chickpeas supply more than 20 per cent of the world with protein and it's one of the earliest cultivated legume crops around the Mediterranean. They are simply delicious!

Blanch the spinach in a pot of boiling water just until wilted, then drain and set aside to cool. Once cool, squeeze to remove the excess liquid.

In the meantime, heat the olive oil in a frying pan and add the onion, garlic, turmeric, coriander, cumin and chilli. Sauté the mixture for 1–2 minutes, then add the tomato paste. Mix well, then add the chopped tomatoes and cook until soft, then add the cooked chickpeas.

Finally, add the cooked spinach and salt to taste, and stir well. Top with the yoghurt and mint. Serve hot.

MUSHROOM AND FARRO STEW

SERVES **4** • PREPARATION TIME **10 MINUTES** • COOKING TIME **1 HOUR**

285 g (10 oz) whole grain farro (soak overnight if you want to reduce the cooking time)

1 onion, finely diced

2 tablespoons olive oil

220 g (8 oz) mixed mushrooms, sliced

2 garlic cloves, finely chopped

1 handful thyme and oregano leaves, chopped

2 tablespoons lemon juice

2 tablespoons parmesan or pecorino cheese, grated

salt and freshly ground black pepper

This hearty mushroom dish is simple to make and healthy to eat. Farro is highly nutritious and filling. It is high in protein, fibre, iron, magnesium and B vitamins. It has a delicious nutty flavour that complements mushrooms.

Half fill a medium saucepan with water. Season with a pinch of salt. Bring to the boil. Add the farro and turn the heat down once it comes back to a boil. Simmer until the farro is tender but still chewy, about 40 minutes if it hasn't been soaked before cooking. Drain and set aside.

In a frying pan, heat the oil to a medium heat, add the onion and sauté for 5 minutes until soft. Add the mushrooms and sauté for 4 minutes. Add the garlic and herbs and continue to sauté for another 2 minutes or until the mushrooms have dropped their juices.

Stir in the cooked farro and lemon juice. Cook for 3 to 5 minutes until heated through.

Stir in the cheese and season with salt and pepper. Serve immediately.

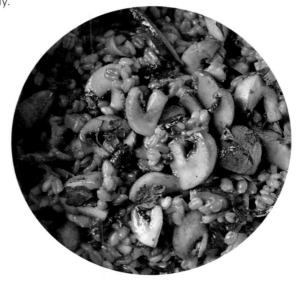

BEETROOT AND YOGHURT

SERVES **2**
PREPARATION TIME **5 MINUTES**
COOKING TIME **20 MINUTES**

2 large beetroots (beets)
2 teaspoons extra-virgin olive oil
12 spinach leaves, chopped
2 thin slices of red onion
salt and freshly ground black pepper
2 tablespoons low-fat Greek yoghurt

A huge range of vegetables can be lightly boiled, steamed or blanched. These include root vegetables, snow peas (mangetout), kale, green beans, broccoli, asparagus, zucchini (courgette), cabbage, peas – it's a huge list.

Cook the beetroots in a pot of boiling water until softened, about 20 minutes. Peel and dice the beetroots when cool enough to handle. Place in a bowl then drizzle with olive oil and sprinkle with the spinach and red onion. Season with salt and pepper and spoon over the yoghurt. Serve hot or warm.

GREEN BEANS AND ALMONDS

SERVES **4**
PREPARATION TIME **5 MINUTES**
COOKING TIME **4 MINUTES**

400 g (14 oz) green beans, trimmed
20 g (¾ oz) slivered almonds
2 teaspoons extra-virgin olive oil
squeeze of lemon juice
salt and freshly ground black pepper

Bring a pot of salted water to the boil. Drop in the green beans and cook for 3–4 minutes until just done. Drain and add the almonds, olive oil and lemon juice. Season with salt and pepper and serve hot or warm.

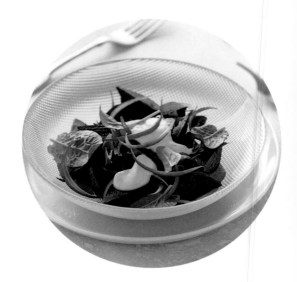

ROAST PUMPKIN SALAD

SERVES **4** · PREPARATION TIME **15 MINUTES** · COOKING TIME **20 MINUTES**

1 teaspoon dried mint

1 teaspoon ground cumin

1 teaspoon ground ginger

½ teaspoon chilli flakes

½ teaspoon ground cinnamon

½ teaspoon cumin seeds

3 tablespoons extra-virgin olive oil

salt and freshly ground black pepper

500 g (1 lb 2 oz) pumpkin (winter squash), peeled, deseeded and thinly sliced

Studies suggest that cinnamon has potential anti-diabetic effects. Some of its extracts not only possess antioxidant and anti-inflammatory properties, but also seem to improve symptoms associated with metabolic syndrome. This spice also has a mild blood cholesterol-lowering effect.

Preheat the oven to 180°C (350°F).

Add the mint, cumin and ginger to a mortar with the chilli flakes, cinnamon and cumin. Pound with the pestle for a few minutes. Transfer to a small bowl and add the olive oil and some salt and pepper. Mix well.

Place the sliced pumpkin on a baking tray and rub with the spiced marinade. Drizzle over any remaining mixture, then roast for 20 minutes.

VARIATIONS

Replace the pumpkin with sweet potato slices.

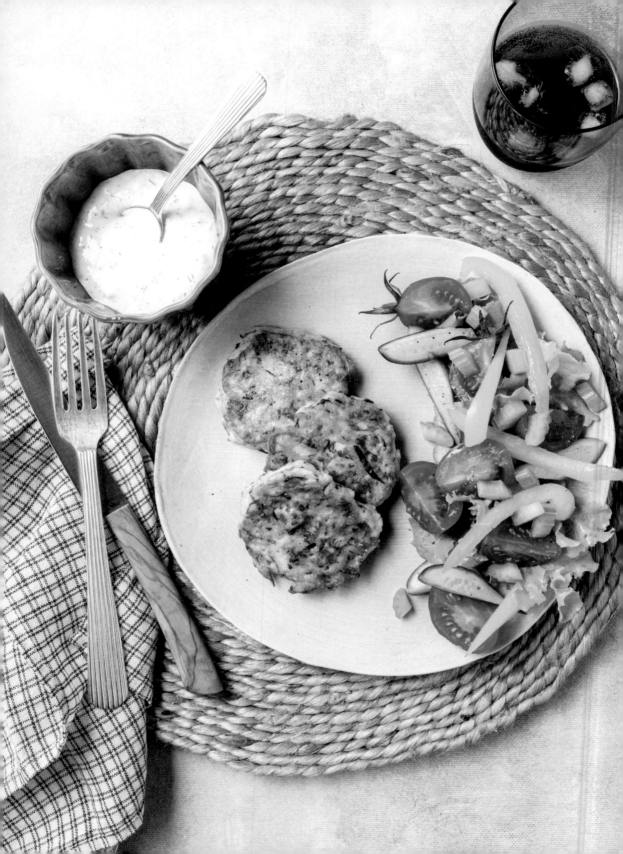

GREEK-STYLE FRITTERS

MAKES **8** • PREPARATION TIME **30 MINUTES** • COOKING TIME **10–20 MINUTES**

1 large zucchini
(courgette)

1 tablespoon chopped
dill

grated zest and juice
of 1 lemon

1 large free-range egg

50 g (1¾ oz) self-
raising flour

40 g (1½ oz)
feta cheese, or
mozzarella cheese

1 tablespoon olive oil

These simple fritters are ready in no time and can be served with almost any salad. It's important to squeeze out the moisture in the grated zucchini (courgette) so the fritters will be firm and not soggy.

Grate the zucchini into a sieve. Press with the back of a spoon to remove the moisture. Put the grated zucchini in a medium bowl. Add the dill, lemon zest and egg and mix well, then add the flour and stir to combine. Add the feta or mozzarella cheese and mix again.

Heat a non-stick frying pan over a medium heat and add the olive oil. Spoon about 1½ tablespoons of mixture into the pan to make individual fritters. Fry for 3 minutes per side, or until golden brown, then squeeze over the lemon juice. You may need to fry them in batches. Serve the fritters with a salad.

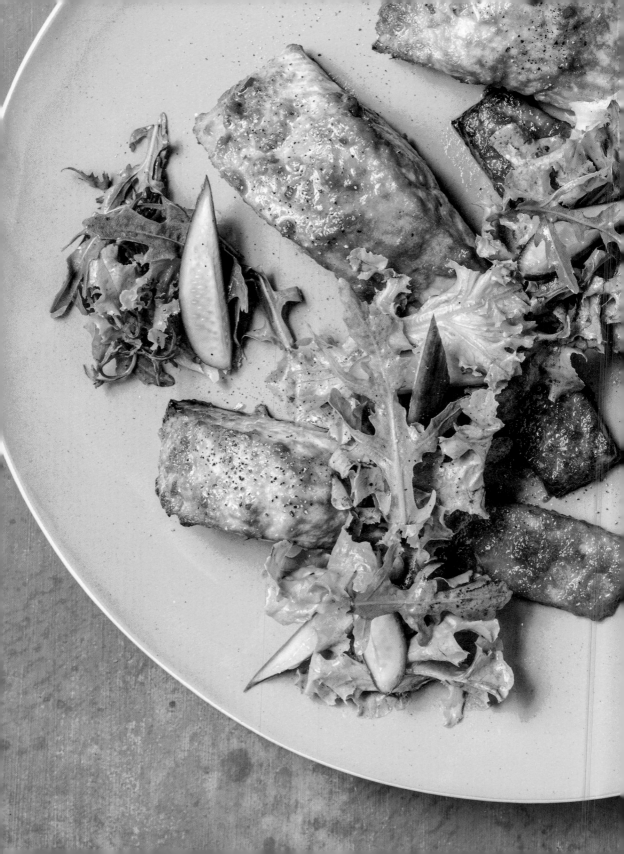

FISH

HONEY-GLAZED SALMON

SERVES **2** • PREPARATION TIME **MARINATING 1 HOUR, THEN 10 MINUTES**
COOKING TIME **15 MINUTES**

300 g (10½ oz) skinless salmon fillets

juice of ½ lemon

MARINADE

1 teaspoon finely chopped ginger

1 garlic clove, finely chopped

½ teaspoon finely chopped red chilli

1 tablespoon olive oil

2 tablespoons soy sauce

1 tablespoon dijon mustard

1 tablespoon honey

Oily fish is an excellent food for dampening the effects of inflammation and high triglycerides. Salmon, especially wild-caught, is rich in omega-3 fatty acids and these fatty acids can help protect us from heart disease.

Prepare the marinade by combining the ginger, garlic, chilli, olive oil and soy sauce. Mix well and add mustard and honey, mixing to a smooth cream.

Place the salmon in a bowl and use half of the marinade to cover the salmon on both sides. Cover and let the salmon marinate in the refrigerator for at least 60 minutes. Set the remaining marinade aside.

Preheat the oven to 190°C (375°F). Place the salmon on a baking tray. Brush with some of the remaining marinade and cook on one side for about 7–8 minutes, then turn over the fish and brush again with marinade and cook for an additional 6–7 minutes, or until done, which will depend on the thickness of the pieces. Squeeze over the lemon juice.

Serve with one or two vegetable dishes or salads.

GRILLED SARDINES
WITH ORANGE, GARLIC AND SPANISH PAPRIKA

SERVES **4** • PREPARATION TIME **MARINATING 30 MINUTES, THEN 10 MINUTES**
COOKING TIME **10 MINUTES**

60 ml (2 fl oz/¼ cup) fresh orange juice

3 garlic cloves, crushed

1 teaspoon smoked red paprika

½ teaspoon ground coriander

¼ teaspoon ground cumin

½ teaspoon freshly ground black pepper

12 fresh sardines, cleaned and gutted

salt, to taste

3 tablespoons chopped flat-leaf (Italian) parsley

Sardines are a popular fish in the Mediterranean. It's plentiful and cheap as well as high in omega-3, iron and vitamin B12.

Combine the orange juice, garlic, paprika and spices in a large bowl and whisk well to combine. Place the sardines in the marinade, turning the fish to ensure they are evenly coated. Cover and set aside to marinate for 30 minutes in the fridge.

Remove the sardines from the marinade. Heat a chargrill pan or barbecue chargrill plate and cook the sardines on one side for 2–3 minutes. Turn the sardines over and cook for another 1–2 minutes, or until cooked through.

Transfer the sardines to a platter and season with salt. Sprinkle with chopped parsley and serve with a salad or cooked vegetables and a slice of wholemeal bread.

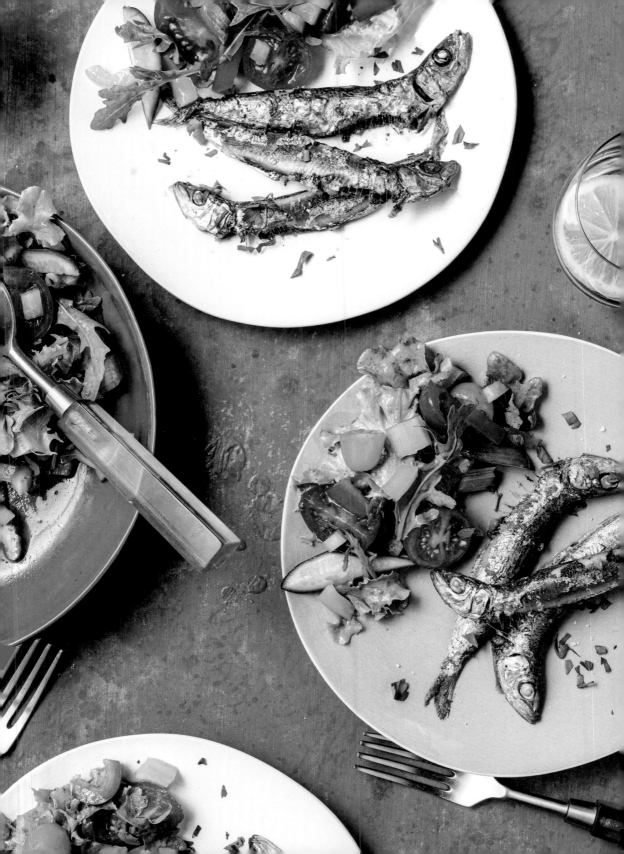

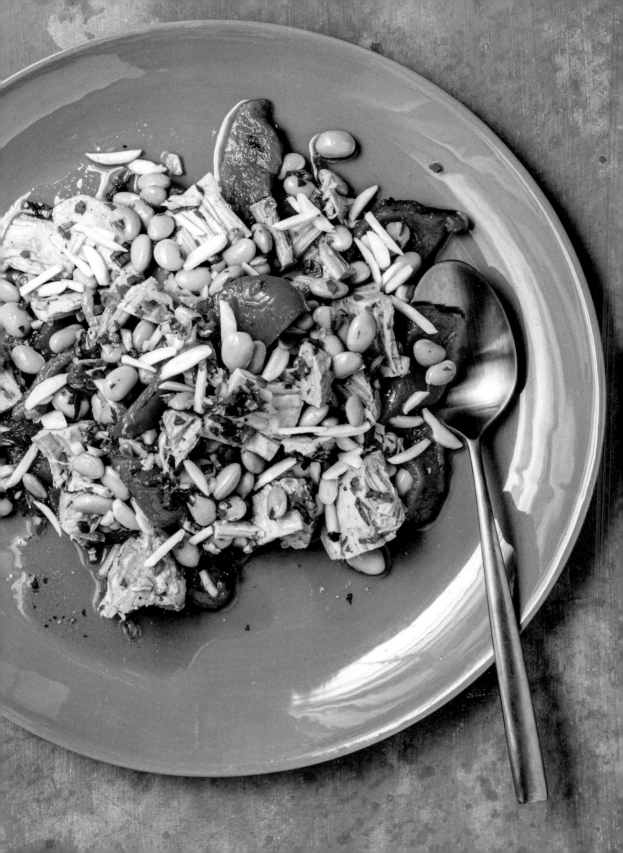

TUNA STEAKS WITH GRILLED CAPSICUM AND EDAMAME SALAD

SERVES **2** • PREPARATION TIME **MARINATING 1 HOUR, THEN 20 MINUTES**
COOKING TIME **35 MINUTES**

300 g (10½ oz) tuna
steaks

60 ml (2 fl oz/¼ cup)
fresh orange juice

300 g (10½ oz)
long red or green
capsicums (bell
peppers)

100 g (3½ oz)
edamame

½ large jalapeño
chilli, or ½ small
hot red chilli

2 tablespoons extra-
virgin olive oil

1 tablespoon finely
sliced flat-leaf
(Italian) parsley

2 garlic cloves,
crushed

juice of ½ lemon

salt and freshly
ground black pepper

2 tablespoons
low-salt soy sauce

2 spring onions
(scallions),
finely sliced

wasabi, to taste

50 g (1¾ oz) slivered
almonds, to serve

Edamame are whole, immature soy beans and some studies
have shown that soy beans may lower circulating cholesterol
levels.

Marinate the tuna in the orange juice for 60 minutes. Turn the fish
after 30 minutes.

In the meantime, heat a chargrill pan or barbecue chargrill plate
over a high heat and grill the capsicums for 10 minutes, turning
frequently, until they're blistered and tender. Peel the skin off and
remove the seeds before chopping them into small dice.

Boil the edamame for 5 minutes in plenty of water. Drain and
place in a small bowl with the jalapeño. Add the olive oil, parsley,
garlic and lemon juice. Stir well and season to taste with salt
and pepper.

In another small bowl, mix the soy sauce with the sliced onion
and a tiny piece of wasabi. Mix well.

Remove the tuna steaks from the orange juice. Heat a non-
stick frying pan with a lid over a medium heat. Place the steaks
in the pan and reduce the heat to low. Cover and cook for up
to 20 minutes, or until just cooked through (depending on the
thickness of the steaks). Remove from the pan and brush with the
soy sauce mix and set aside to cool.

To serve, break the tuna into bite-sized chunks and place in a
serving dish, add the capsicum, edamame and jalapeño along
with the dressing and toss. Sprinkle with almonds.

SAUTÉED GREENS
WITH BROWN RICE AND TUNA

SERVES **2** • PREPARATION TIME **10 MINUTES** • COOKING TIME **25 MINUTES**

65 g (2¼ oz/⅓ cup) brown rice

2 tablespoons extra-virgin olive oil

100 g (3½ oz) tuna steak

1 brown onion, finely chopped

1 garlic clove, finely chopped

1 zucchini (courgette), chopped

1 broccoli head, florets chopped

155 g (5½ oz/1 cup) peas

125 ml (4 fl oz/½ cup) vegetable stock

100 g (3½ oz/2 cups) baby spinach

1 tablespoon toasted sesame seeds, to serve

A sprinkling of fresh or toasted nuts or seeds for added crunch is great with any salad. Choose from pepitas (pumpkin seeds), sesame seeds, linseeds (flax seeds), almonds, walnuts, Brazil nuts, and many others.

The natural carbohydrates and fibre in brown rice make this a sustaining dish. Add a small amount of fish and you have great protein and good fats that will help keep you satisfied all day.

Add the rice to a saucepan, cover with 170 ml (5½ fl oz/⅔ cup) water and bring to the boil. Cover with a lid, reduce the heat to a simmer and cook for 25 minutes, or until tender. Drain well and set aside until needed.

While the rice is cooking, heat 1 tablespoon of the oil in a small frying pan until very hot. Sear the tuna in the pan until just done, about 1–2 minutes on each side depending on the thickness of the tuna. Cut into 2.5 cm (1 in) cubes. Set aside.

Heat the remaining oil in a clean frying pan over a medium–high heat. Add the onion and garlic, then lower the heat to medium and sauté for 5–6 minutes, or until the onion has softened and browned. Add the zucchini, broccoli and peas to the pan and cook, stirring, for 2 minutes, then lower the heat, pour over the vegetable stock and cook for a further 4–5 minutes, or until the vegetables are tender. Stir in the spinach and cooked brown rice, to heat through, then remove from the heat and divide between bowls.

To serve, top with the tuna and sprinkle with sesame seeds.

VARIATIONS

You can replace the tuna with any other fish you like, or even hard-boiled eggs or tofu.

WHITE FISH WITH GREEK SALAD

SERVES **4** · PREPARATION TIME **10 MINUTES** · COOKING TIME **10 MINUTES**

2 tomatoes, diced

1 Lebanese cucumber, diced

1 red onion, finely sliced

½ teaspoon dried oregano

40 g (1½ oz) pitted black olives

4 tablespoons roughly chopped flat-leaf (Italian) parsley

2 tablespoons extra-virgin olive oil

juice of ½ lemon

60 g (2 oz) feta cheese, crumbled

4 × 180–200 g (6½–7 oz) white fish fillets, skin on

Greek salad is known the world over, but what a simple salad it is to complement fish.

Combine the tomato, cucumber, onion, oregano, olives and parsley in a serving bowl. Drizzle with 1 tablespoon of the olive oil and the lemon juice and toss together. Add the feta to the salad.

Heat a large non-stick frying pan over a high heat and add the remaining oil. Cook the fillets, skin side down, for 3–5 minutes, then carefully turn over and cook for another 3–5 minutes on the other side, gently moving the pan occasionally to ensure the skin doesn't stick. Serve the fish with the salad.

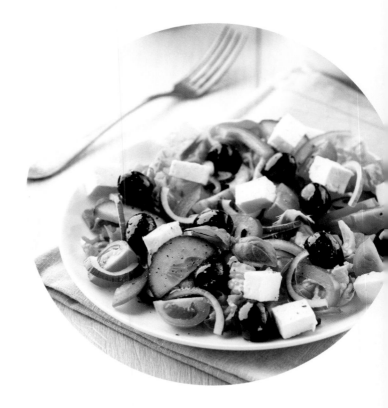

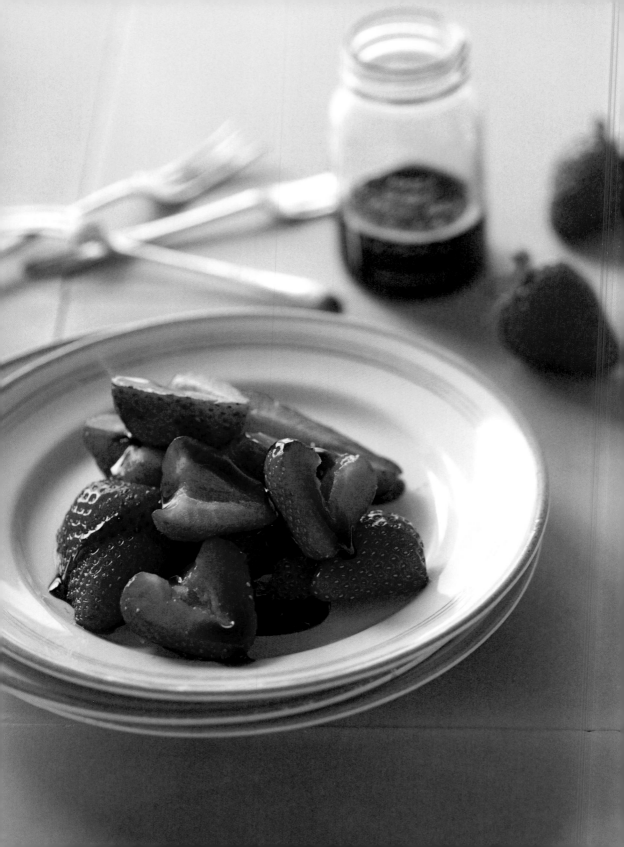

DESSERTS

BALSAMIC STRAWBERRIES

SERVES **2** · PREPARATION TIME **5 MINUTES**

250 g (9 oz/1⅔ cups) strawberries, hulled

1 tablespoon balsamic vinegar

2 tablespoons low-fat Greek-style yoghurt

It's becoming increasingly clear that what we eat affects the vitality and health of our skin, and how quickly it ages. Cherries, blueberries, blackcurrants, strawberries, plums and apples are low-glycaemic fruits rich in vitamins and phytochemicals that possess skin-protecting properties. They are instrumental in keeping our skin glowing, smooth and clear. Eating a variety of fruits daily that are rich in carotenoids, lutein and zeaxanthin improves skin tone and luminance, and protects against UV-induced redness and photo-ageing.

Fruits rich in carotenoids are papaya, watermelon, rockmelon (cantaloupe), mangoes and oranges, while excellent sources of lutein and zeaxanthin are kiwi fruit, grapes and oranges.

The benefits of regularly consuming fruit are not limited to skin health. At the end of a meal, replacing the usual energy-dense sweet and fatty dessert or ice cream with a fruit salad is one of the best strategies for keeping your body weight at bay while promoting metabolic health. Tropical fruit salads could include mango, papaya and rockmelon with a passionfruit topping and the juice of an orange as the sauce. Winter salads could include chopped apples, pears and a mix of berries like strawberries, blueberries and raspberries also with an orange juice sauce.

Place the strawberries in a large mixing bowl. Drizzle with the vinegar and mix gently. Serve with the yoghurt.

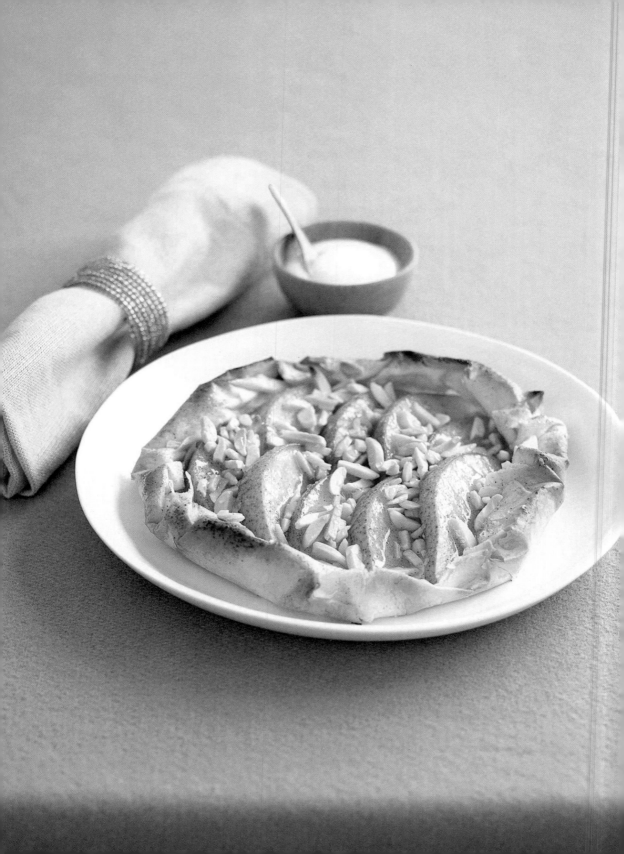

HONEY PEARS

1 tablespoon honey
4 beurre bosc pears, halved and cored
2 cinnamon sticks
4 long pieces orange rind

This is a warming winter treat that is simple to make and delicious to eat.

Preheat the oven to 200°C (400°F).

Combine the honey and 250 ml (8½ fl oz/ 1 cup) cold water in a roasting tin. Add the pears, skin side up. Add the cinnamon and orange rind and cover the pan tightly with aluminium foil.

Roast for 30 minutes, then remove the foil and turn the pears, basting them with the juice. Roast for another 30 minutes, or until the pears are caramelised and tender.

PEAR OR APPLE FILO TART

12 sheets filo pastry
2 tablespoons light olive oil
2 large apples or pears, thinly sliced
2 tablespoons honey
1 teaspoon ground cardamom
30 g (1 oz/¼ cup) slivered almonds

Paper-thin sheets of filo pastry have no fat, unlike other pastries, but they still give a satisfying crunch.

Preheat the oven to 200°C (400°F).

Line a large baking tray with baking paper. On a work bench, spread out 1 sheet of filo pastry. Using a pastry brush, brush the filo with a little oil, then top with another filo sheet and brush with oil. Repeat with a third sheet of filo.

Fold the sheets in half and top with one-quarter of the fruit. Drizzle with one-quarter of the honey and sprinkle with one-quarter of the cardamom. Fold up the sides of the filo to cover the outside edges of the fruit. Lift onto the baking tray.

Repeat with remaining filo and fruit to make four tarts. Brush the tarts lightly with oil and sprinkle with almonds. Bake the tarts for about 8–10 minutes, or until crisp and golden.

POACHED PEACHES

SERVES **4**
PREPARATION TIME **10 MINUTES**
COOKING TIME **20 MINUTES**

425 ml (14½ fl oz) sweet white wine, or water

2 tablespoons honey

1 vanilla bean, split lengthways and seeds scraped

4 large ripe peaches

Place the wine, honey and vanilla bean and seeds in a saucepan large enough to hold all the peaches, then gently heat until the honey has dissolved. Lower the peaches into the pan, cover and simmer gently for 15–20 minutes until just tender. Turn the fruit while cooking.

Remove the cooked peaches from the pan and set to one side in a bowl to cool. If the skin hasn't already come off, it will peel off easily now. You can reduce the cooking liquid a little, or just pour it over the peaches as is and refrigerate until you want to serve. The liquid will keep them moist. Serve at room temperature.

GRILLED PEACHES OR APRICOTS

SERVES **4**
PREPARATION TIME **10 MINUTES**
COOKING TIME **30 MINUTES**

4 peaches or 8 apricots, halved

2 teaspoons honey (optional)

This is such a simple recipe and the fruit is delicious served hot.

Preheat the oven to 200°C (400°F).

Line a large baking tray with baking paper. Place the halved peaches on the tray, skin side down. Drizzle with the honey. Bake for 20–30 minutes or until tender. Serve.

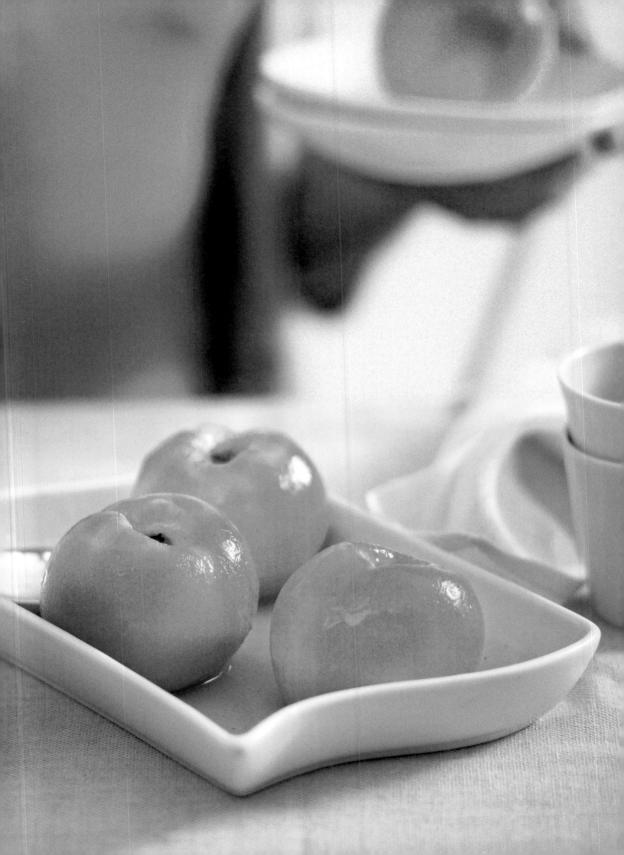

SIDES, SNACKS & DIPS

SPICY ROASTED CHICKPEAS

SERVES **4** • PREPARATION TIME **SOAKING OVERNIGHT, THEN 10 MINUTES**
COOKING TIME **2 HOURS**

425 g (15 oz) dried chickpeas

1 tablespoon extra-virgin olive oil

1 teaspoon ground cumin

1 teaspoon chilli powder

½ teaspoon cayenne pepper

salt, to taste

Simple and tasty, these spicy chickpeas are a great snack to keep on hand or to add to a veggie bowl.

Soak the chickpeas overnight. Drain the chickpeas, place in a large saucepan and cover with water. Bring to the boil, then simmer for about 45 minutes to 1 hour until cooked but still firm.

Drain and rinse the chickpeas, then pat dry with paper towel. The drier you get them, the crunchier they'll be.

Preheat the oven to 200°C (400°F).

To a bowl, add the chickpeas, olive oil, cumin, chilli powder, cayenne pepper and salt. Toss well to coat evenly.

Spread the chickpeas out on a baking tray lined with baking paper and roast for 15–20 minutes. Toss the chickpeas, then continue roasting for an additional 15–20 minutes, or until browned. Turn off the oven and leave the chickpeas inside to cool. They will continue to cook and dry out without burning. Leave them in the oven until they are cold, even overnight.

The chickpeas should remain crispy stored for about 5 days in an airtight container.

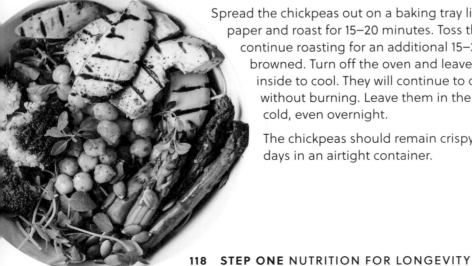

BAKED NUT AND LEGUME NUTRIENT BALLS

MAKES **4** • PREPARATION TIME **SOAKING OVERNIGHT, THEN 20 MINUTES**
COOKING TIME **1 HOUR 5 MINUTES**

60 g (2 oz) dried chickpeas

100 g (3½ oz) red lentils

30 g (1 oz) brown rice

75 g (2¾ oz/1¼ cups) broccoli, finely chopped

½ red capsicum (bell pepper), deseeded and finely chopped

1 celery stalk, finely chopped

25 g (1 oz) pepitas (pumpkin seeds)

25 g (1 oz) sunflower kernels

1 teaspoon thyme leaves

50 g (1¾ oz/⅓ cup) almonds

150 g (5½ oz) cashew nuts

½ teaspoon tamari

1 teaspoon brown miso paste

1 tablespoon sesame seeds, to coat

These balls make delicious savoury snacks.

Soak the chickpeas overnight, then drain and rinse under cold water. Bring 300 ml (10 fl oz) water to the boil in a small saucepan and add the chickpeas. Bring back to the boil, cover and simmer for 45 minutes, or until the chickpeas are soft but not soggy – they should have some bite. Drain and set aside.

Rinse the lentils and place them in another saucepan with 300 ml (10 fl oz) boiling water. Bring back to the boil, cover and simmer for 20 minutes, or until soft. Drain and set aside.

Place the rice in a small saucepan and cover well with water. Add a little salt and bring to the boil. Simmer for about 30 minutes, or until really soft. Drain and set aside.

Combine the rice, broccoli, capsicum, celery, seeds and thyme in a large bowl.

Preheat the oven to 180°C (350°F).

Put the chickpeas, lentils, nuts, tamari and miso in a food processor and blitz until you obtain a rough paste (not a smooth purée). Add this mixture to the rice mix, combine well and season to taste.

Roll the mixture into small balls with your hands. Gently roll the balls in the sesame seeds to coat. Place on a baking tray lined with baking paper and bake the balls for 20 minutes, or until golden brown.

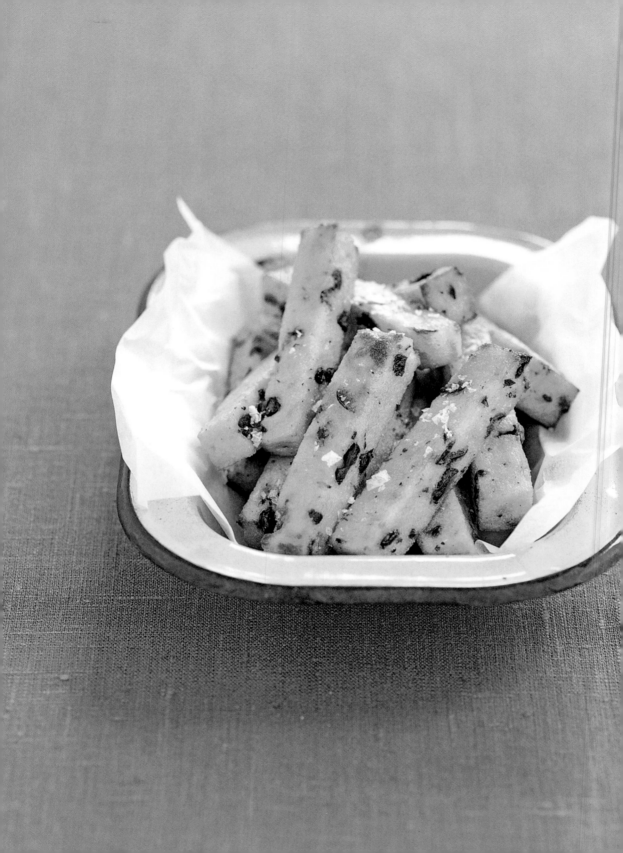

POLENTA CHIPS

SERVES **4** • PREPARATION TIME **10 MINUTES** • COOKING TIME **40 MINUTES**

150 g (5½ oz/1 cup) polenta (not quick-cooking)

¾ teaspoon salt

1 garlic clove, crushed

1 teaspoon chopped sage

1 teaspoon chopped rosemary

10 black olives, pitted and chopped

1 tablespoon extra-virgin olive oil

grated parmesan cheese, to serve

Polenta is a filling and satisfying snack, and these herbs of the Lamiaceae family – peppermint, sage, rosemary, spearmint, thyme – contain a powerful antioxidant.

Combine the polenta with 750 ml (25½ fl oz/3 cups) water and the salt in a heavy-based saucepan and bring to the boil over a medium heat, whisking as it heats. Reduce the heat to low–medium and cook, stirring constantly with a long-handled wooden spoon, until the polenta begins to pull away from the side of the pan, about 15–20 minutes. Remove from the heat and stir in the garlic, herbs and olives.

Oil a baking tray with the olive oil then transfer the cooked polenta to the tray, spreading it out evenly with a dampened rubber spatula to form a 1 cm (½ in) thick layer. Refrigerate for 2–3 hours until firm.

Preheat the oven to 200°C (400°F). Remove the polenta from the fridge, turn it out of the tray onto a clean surface and cut into long rectangular sticks about 8.5 × 2 cm (3¼ × ¾ in).

Place the chips on a large baking tray lined with baking paper and bake for 15–20 minutes, turning halfway during cooking, or until golden.

Serve lightly dusted with grated parmesan cheese.

HOME-MADE TAHINI DIP

SERVES **4** • PREPARATION TIME **5 MINUTES** • COOKING TIME **2–3 MINUTES**

45 g (1½ oz) sesame seeds

1 tablespoon extra-virgin olive oil

¼ teaspoon ground cumin

2 garlic cloves

1 teaspoon lemon juice

salt, to taste

Sesame seeds are also called the 'seeds of longevity'; they are considered to be the oldest oilseed crop known to humanity. These tiny, super tasty seeds can be used whole in salads or ground into tahini. Unhulled sesame seeds are more nutrient-rich and have a toasty, smoky flavour. Sesame seeds contain several specific antioxidant compounds. Sesamin is associated with reduced serum levels of cholesterol.

Toast the sesame seeds in a dry frying pan over a high heat for a few minutes until golden. Be careful not to burn them.

Combine the toasted seeds with the olive oil in a small food processor or blender and blend to a paste. Add the cumin, garlic, lemon juice and keep blending. Taste and adjust the lemon juice and add salt as needed. You may need to add a little water to make a smooth paste.

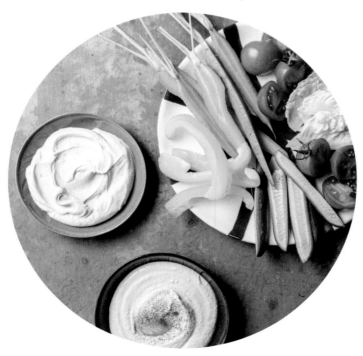

HOME-MADE HUMMUS

SERVES **4** • PREPARATION TIME **10 MINUTES**

500 g (1 lb 2 oz) cooked chickpeas (see pages 130–131)

60 ml (2 fl oz/¼ cup) Home-made tahini dip (page 122)

2 large garlic cloves, chopped

juice of 2 lemons

1 tablespoon extra-virgin olive oil, plus extra for drizzling

salt, to taste

½ teaspoon smoked paprika

2 tablespoons chopped flat-leaf (Italian) parsley

Hummus is one of the most versatile and tasty dips eaten all around the Mediterranean. I love it!

Place the chickpeas, tahini, garlic, lemon juice and olive oil in a food processor and blend until you have a smooth and creamy purée. Add a little water if needed to loosen and season with salt.

To serve the hummus, drizzle with the extra olive oil, some smoked paprika and the chopped parsley.

Hummus tastes best if made a day in advance and then served. Use on sandwiches as a spread or use as a dip for celery, carrots, cucumbers or zucchini (courgette).

VARIATIONS

Add 1 roasted and peeled red capsicum (bell pepper), ½ teaspoon ground cumin and ½ teaspoon cayenne pepper to the blender. Or add 2 tablespoons finely chopped olives and 1 tablespoon of capers to the finished hummus.

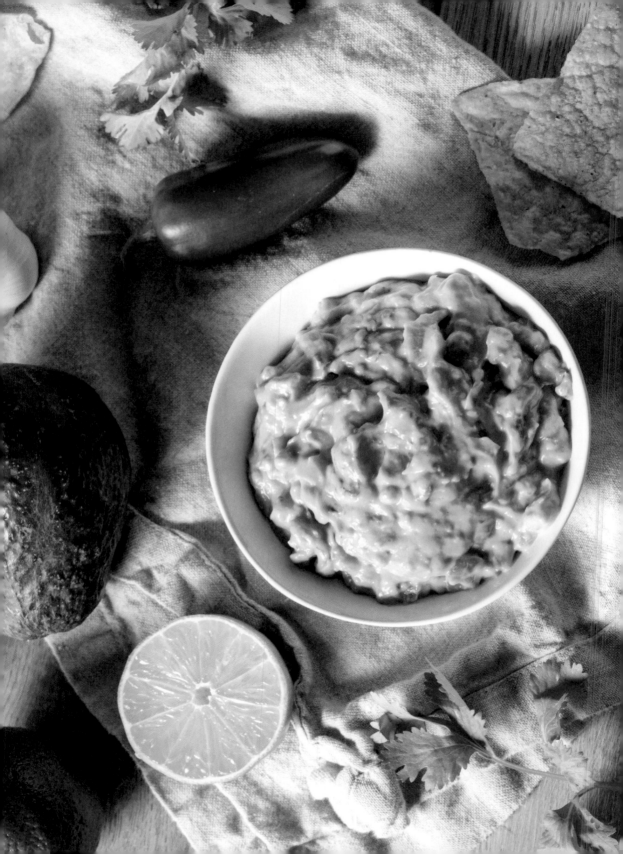

HOME-MADE GUACAMOLE

3 ripe avocados, halved, stones removed

½ small onion, finely diced

1 garlic clove, minced

½ red or green capsicum (bell pepper), finely diced

salt, to taste

juice of 1 lime, or ½ lemon

3 tablespoons finely chopped coriander (cilantro)

Guacamole serves up plenty of health benefits, specifically the monounsaturated fats in avocados that play an important role in maintaining healthy cholesterol levels. Avocados also contain as many as twenty different vitamins and minerals.

Scoop out the avocado flesh into a bowl and mash with a fork. Make it as chunky or smooth as you like. Add the onion, garlic and capsicum, and mix well. Then add some salt, lime juice to taste and the coriander, and mix well.

VARIATIONS

You can add 1 ripe but firm diced tomato, and/or 1 jalapeño chilli, seeds removed and finely diced.

EGGPLANT DIP

SERVES **4** · PREPARATION TIME **30 MINUTES** · COOKING TIME **1 HOUR**

750 g (1 lb 11 oz) eggplants (aubergines)

700 g (1 lb 9 oz) ripe tomatoes

2 tablespoons extra-virgin olive oil, plus 1 extra teaspoon to serve

1 tablespoon crushed garlic

¾ teaspoon ground cumin

½ teaspoon sweet paprika

¼ teaspoon cayenne pepper

2 tablespoons finely chopped coriander (cilantro)

2 tablespoons lemon juice

salt, to taste

Eggplant (aubergine) is a really versatile vegetable. It can be baked, barbecued, stuffed, puréed, curried and pickled.

Pierce each eggplant in several places with a knife. Halve each eggplant lengthways.

Preheat a chargrill pan or barbecue chargrill plate over a high heat, then grill the eggplants until the skins have blackened and the flesh is tender (about 20 minutes depending on the heat). Place the hot eggplant in a colander. While still hot, carefully peel the skin off, then allow the flesh to drain until cool. Squeeze gently to remove any remaining juices.

Using a grater, coarsely grate the tomatoes until you are left with just the skins, which you can discard. Meanwhile, heat the olive oil in a non-stick frying pan over a medium heat. Add the garlic, cumin, paprika and cayenne pepper, and then the tomatoes. Cook for 15–20 minutes, or until the sauce thickens.

Mash the eggplant flesh with a fork and add to the pan. Stir in the chopped coriander and continue cooking, stirring often, until thick and juicy, about 10–15 minutes. Transfer to a bowl and add the lemon juice and salt to taste.

You can eat this warm or cold. Store covered in the fridge for up to 3 days. Before serving, return the dip to room temperature and toss with 1 teaspoon olive oil.

CASHEW CREAM DIP

SERVES **4**
PREPARATION TIME **2 HOURS SOAKING,
PLUS 5–10 MINUTES**

280 g (10 oz) raw cashew nuts

2 tablespoons nutritional yeast

2 tablespoons extra-virgin olive oil

juice of 1½ large lemons

1 teaspoon white miso (optional)

½ garlic clove, minced (optional)

1 teaspoon dried marjoram, or 1 tablespoon finely chopped flat-leaf (Italian) parsley (optional)

salt, to taste

A delicious dip that is creamy, but made without any dairy products. It can be swirled through soup just as you would add sour cream.

Put the cashews in a bowl and cover with at least 3 cm (1¼ in) cold water. Soak for at least 2 hours, then rinse well and drain.

Blend the cashews, yeast, olive oil, lemon juice and 125 ml (4 fl oz/½ cup) water in a food processor until creamy. Stop to scrape down the sides every few minutes. Taste and adjust the flavour as needed, adding more salt, nutritional yeast for a cheesy taste, and lemon juice for acidity.

The dip can be served plain, or you can add the miso, garlic and marjoram for a tastier flavour.

Use this cream as a dip, a spread or a filling for ravioli or lasagne. Store covered in the fridge for up to 5 days.

HERBED TZATZIKI DIP

SERVES **2**
PREPARATION TIME **5 MINUTES**

250 g (9 oz/1 cup) low-fat Greek-style yoghurt

1 small cucumber, grated

1 garlic clove, crushed

2 tablespoons lemon juice

1 teaspoon finely chopped dill

4–5 basil leaves, chopped

1 small jalapeño, seeds removed and minced (optional)

1 tablespoon extra-virgin olive oil (optional)

salt and freshly ground black pepper

Whether you use mint or basil, both are from the mint family and will add a fresh taste to this light summery dip.

Place all of the ingredients in a mixing bowl and stir to combine. Taste and adjust the seasoning.

TIPS

If it is a small cucumber, do not remove the skin, but for a large one, I suggest peeling it, then cutting the cucumber in half lengthways and removing the seeds with a spoon.

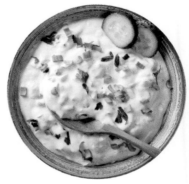

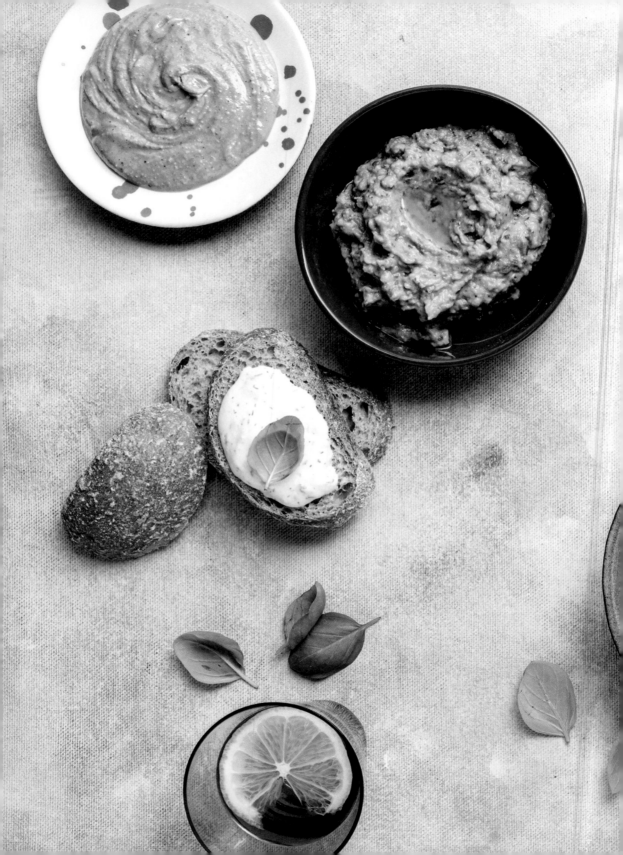

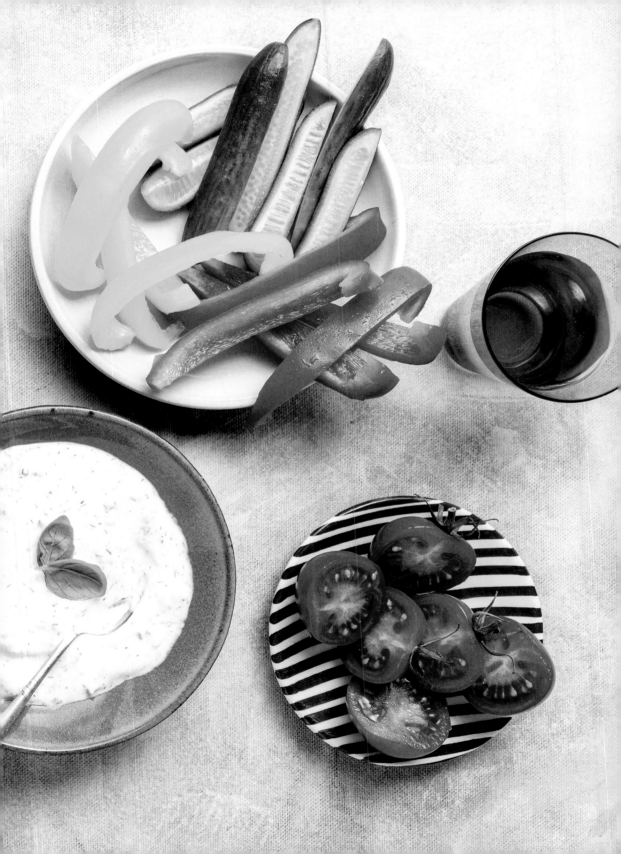

BASICS

BEANS AND LEGUMES

Always have a variety of whole grains and legumes in your cupboard. Unlike many other food products, they will last for several months stored at room temperature and in dark conditions.

To keep a steady supply of beans, lentils or chickpeas on hand, cover a cup of your choice of legume with plenty of water and set it aside to soak overnight. Soaking reduces the production of excessive gas and bloating in our gut but more importantly it helps to remove toxins in dried beans. Beans that have been soaked will cook more evenly and quickly. Always discard the soaking water. Then, the next day, when you go to the kitchen to cook, put a pot of water on the stove and add the drained legumes. Within an hour or two of simmering, they will be ready to cool and store in glass containers in the fridge, ready to use. Cook brown rice, farro or barley to have on hand too.

Use cooked brown rice or legumes as a side dish for your lunch, or to add to a vegetable soup or stew for dinner. A legume salad with lots of fresh vegetables is a healthy option for lunch or as a side dish for dinner.

COOKING CHICKPEAS AND BEANS

Dried chickpeas and beans triple in size (if not a little more) when cooked, so 220 g (8 oz/1 cup) dried chickpeas will make about 500 g (1 lb 2 oz oz/3 cups) cooked chickpeas.

Add the chickpeas or beans to a large bowl and cover with plenty of water. Soak for 8 hours or overnight. As they rehydrate, the beans absorb the water.

To cook the soaked chickpeas or beans, drain, then add them to a large pot, cover with plenty of water and bring to a boil. Reduce the heat and simmer until tender, about 45 minutes to 2 hours, depending on how old they are.

When simmering, you can keep the lid off or on but slightly ajar (allowing some steam to escape while cooking so they don't boil over). Chickpeas or beans simmered without a lid will be cooked, but firm. Cooked with the lid on, but ajar, they will be creamier, softer and break apart more easily. These are perfect for hummus or dishes where you want to purée them. Add a generous pinch of salt when they are almost cooked, not at the beginning, as salting the beans too early can cause them to become a little tough.

The cooking time can vary a lot depending on size and freshness, so check them every 30 minutes to judge the best cooking time.

Store the cooked beans in an airtight container in the fridge for up to 5 days, or freeze them for several months.

Once you know how to cook dried chickpeas and beans, you'll always have them on hand. They're really easy to make.

COOKING LENTILS

There's no need to soak lentils, split peas or adzuki beans before you cook them. They can take as little as 20 minutes to cook in water.

Bring plenty of water to a gentle boil, reduce the heat and simmer the lentils for about 30 minutes, discarding any foam that rises to the surface.

COOKING FARRO

Farro has a chewy texture and nutty flavour.

First, rinse the dried farro in cold water. Bring a pot of water to the boil and add the farro. Cook until it becomes tender and chewy but still has an al dente bite. The cooking time will vary depending on the age and variety of your farro. When cooked to your liking, drain the grains and run a little cold water through them to stop the cooking. Cooked farro keeps in the fridge for 5 days, but you can freeze it for even longer.

COOKING QUINOA

Quinoa is not actually a grain, but a grain-like seed first grown in South America.

Use 435 ml (15 fl oz/1¾ cups) water for every 200 g (7 oz/1 cup) quinoa. If you use too much water the quinoa can become mushy.

Place the quinoa and water in a medium saucepan and bring to a boil. Cover, then reduce the heat and simmer for 15 minutes. Remove the pan from the heat and let it sit, covered, for another 10 minutes, then remove the lid and fluff up the quinoa with a fork.

STEP TWO

EXERCISE:
A POWERFUL MEDICINE

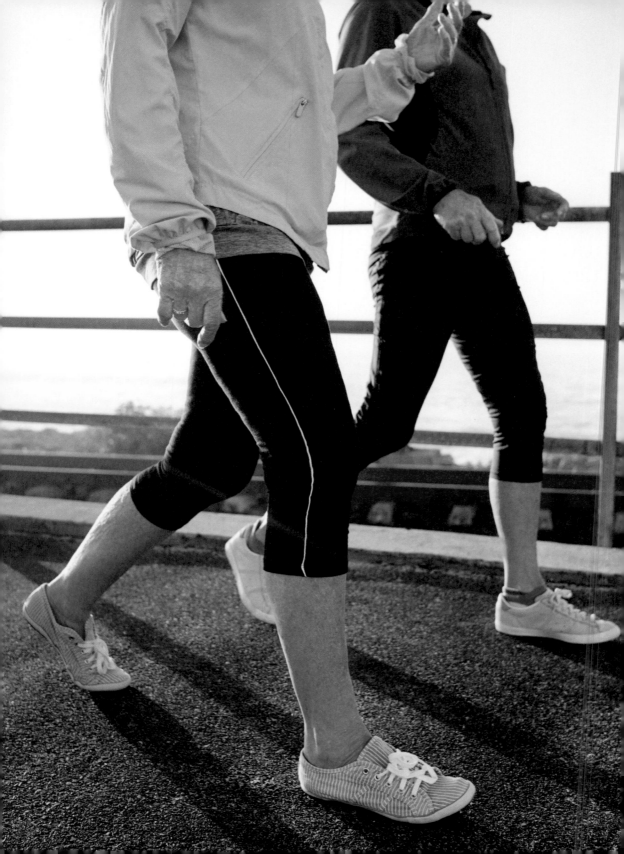

THE IMPORTANCE OF EXERCISE

There are plenty of excellent reasons to be physically active, apart from being fitter and looking good. Much like the air we breathe and the food we eat, movement is essential to our health.

Our bodies have evolved over thousands of years to function optimally with daily physical exertion. Only these days we don't have to walk for hours to bring back firewood or till soil with basic implements to grow enough food to survive. Nevertheless we are metabolically and genetically programmed to operate at our best with constant and regular physical activity.

Physical inactivity is one of the biggest public health problem of the 21st century. How many hours do you sit at a desk each day? What about watching television or looking at a screen for hours? Studies suggest that long periods of inactivity increase the risk of a whole range of health issues, from diabetes, hypertension and cardiovascular disease to cancer and dementia.

The benefits of regular physical activity are reduced risk of heart disease, strokes, cancer and dementia; better control of blood glucose and insulin, which is important especially if you have diabetes or prediabetes; weight control; improvement of depression and anxiety; and potentially a reversal of age-related decline in strength and mobility.

LET'S GET MOVING

Physical activity is basically all the ways in which you move your body on a daily basis. This could include walking to and from the bus stop, cleaning up at home, doing yard work, or standing up from your desk to do a few stretches.

Exercise is what you do intentionally for the purposes of improving your health and fitness, burning calories, building muscle, and learning a physical skill like dance or playing tennis. Effectively, exercise is *planned*, *structured* and *sustained* physical activity.

As for structured exercise, it doesn't necessarily have to take up a lot of your time. Sixty minutes of aerobic exercise (the sort that makes your heart pump faster and breath come quicker) every day is ideal, but even shorter bouts of 10 minutes or so, spread throughout the day, can provide benefits. Then, when the weekend rolls around, take on some longer and more energetic bouts of aerobic exercise or high-intensity interval training (HIIT).

For the most part, physical activity is either free or low cost: truly a wonder-drug for healthy longevity. The challenge of course is that physical activity and exercise require a little more effort than just taking a daily pill. But this regular effort is an investment in your health and healthy longevity: a daily down-payment to help you gain all the benefits of moving better, being fitter and more able in your daily life, feeling better physically and mentally, and avoiding chronic disease, as you age. So much better than ending up on all sorts of medication, or even in hospital, and having no quality of life.

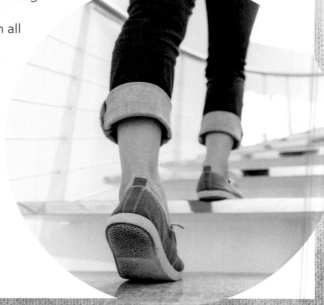

PHYSICAL ACTIVITY

Not only does physical activity throughout your day prevent blood from stagnating (by having your muscles pumping it pushes blood back to your heart to be oxygenated and sent out afresh), you even burn extra calories throughout the day compared to sitting still.

Simple steps you can take are to move your body every waking hour. This could be as simple as fidgeting – moving your body around, bending, twisting, bouncing your legs or feet while sitting – through to standing up from sitting, walking 20–30 paces, or doing some light stretches or strengthening exercises.

Ways to up your physical activity at work:

- Take stairs whenever you get an opportunity.
- If you have to take a phone call, stand up while you're talking.
- If you need to speak to a co-worker, walk to their office.
- Set up a regular 5-minute stretch time with your colleagues.
- For a meeting take a walk with your colleagues instead of sitting in an office.

Ways to up your physical activity at home:

- Do a housework chore like vacuuming, sweeping, dusting, etc.
- Set a timer and stop what you are doing every hour or two and do some stretches.Turn some music on and take a break to sway to the music.
- Do 5 minutes of push-ups, leg lifts or another exercise every hour or so.

> **When you stop exercising regularly it takes only 7 to 10 days for the metabolic and fitness health benefits to significantly decrease.**

REGULAR EXERCISE

OK so now you know you need to be physically active throughout each day, let's talk about regular exercise. Think of exercise as the stimulus that creates lasting positive change in your body – kind of like an upgrade.

There are a few different types of exercise. Exercise that develops your:

- *aerobic* (cardiorespiratory or metabolic) fitness
- *bone* and *muscular* strength and endurance
- *neuromuscular* ability, like balance, posture and coordination
- *flexibility*, like stretching, yoga and tai chi.

All of these are important for optimum benefit and health.

HOW MUCH AND HOW OFTEN?

Guidelines on exercise from the World Health Organization, the US Centers for Disease Control, and the American College of Sports Medicine agree on the following:

- All adults should achieve *at least* 150 minutes per week (150 minutes is half an hour five times a week) of moderate intensity aerobic exercise, or 75 minutes of vigorous intensity aerobic exercise per week (75 minutes is 15 minutes a day five times a week)*.
- Strength training that works all the major muscle groups should be performed at a minimum of two times per week.

*Note that 150 to 300 minutes a week is ideal for moderate intensity aerobic exercise or 75 to 150 minutes of vigorous aerobic exercise a week.

> No matter how old or fit you are everyone should do some strength-training exercises.

BEFORE YOU START

If you've been sedentary, you need to start exercising gradually. Throw yourself into this too fast and you'll end up very sore and possibly injured. Begin slowly – brisk walking is great – then gradually increase the length and frequency of your workout sessions.

If you're older, or have injuries or existing illnesses, check with your doctor or a sports medicine specialist before starting an exercise regimen. They can advise you of any potential health issues and how to proceed.

If you've never had proper instruction in strength training, even if you intend to focus on body-weight exercises, it can be helpful to have some sessions with a personal trainer to ensure you learn the right technique. This is important, too, when starting yoga, tai chi or any martial art – qualified instructors can make sure you are doing it properly and show you the right way.

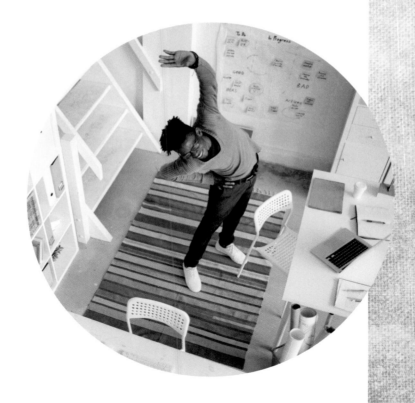

AEROBIC EXERCISE

Aerobic exercise is anything that gets your heart rate up and breathing going while moving your body. This includes walking, jogging, swimming, rowing, cycling, stair climbing – movements which are done repetitively using large muscle groups. When you need to get fitness credits in the bank, the first place to turn is aerobic exercise. It's the sort that improves our cardio-respiratory system – the heart and lungs. Adding it to your routine will grow stocks in both your physical and psychological health.

There are many ways to add aerobic exercise into your routine. These are just some of the moderate-intensity activities that can go towards making up your minimum 150 minutes each week:

- brisk walking
- cycling at less than 16 km/h (10 miles/h)
- water aerobics
- doubles tennis
- volleyball
- ballroom dancing
- gardening or raking the yard.

High-intensity exercise – of which you need at least 75 minutes each week – can be made up of activities like:

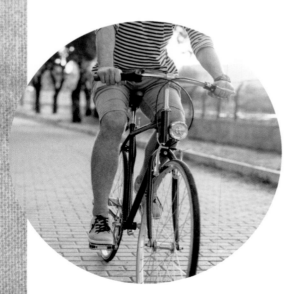

- uphill or race walking
- jogging or running
- stair-walking
- cycling at more than 16 km/h (10 miles/h)
- singles tennis
- strenuous fitness classes
- aerobic dancing
- heavy gardening that involves digging, or hoeing
- jumping rope
- swimming laps.

Most aerobic exercise is rhythmic, repetitive and preferably involves the large muscle groups of your lower body. It also increases your heart rate and breathing rate, both of which help to supply nutrients and oxygen to the body to produce energy and keep the body moving.

Exercise doesn't necessarily need to be boring and it certainly doesn't have to be something you'd rather avoid. In fact, the more activities you find that you really enjoy the easier it will be to integrate more movement and fun into your everyday life.

Need inspiration? You could ...

- Get yourself a bike and go riding whenever you can.
- Convince some of your work friends to go for a walk each lunchtime. You can even sort out a step or time challenge – competition is often good for motivation.
- Take the stairs or run up the escalators.
- When you get up in the morning or home in the evening, put on some of your favourite songs and dance like no one's watching.
- Keep some hand weights near your desk and do some bicep curls and other arm exercises a few times a day.

- Get a dog. Only if it's practical, of course, but they are excellent inspiration for going on long walks, playing and throwing balls.
- Set up an exercise station in front of the TV. It might be a stationary cycle, treadmill or a yoga mat with some resistance bands.
- See if you can get your friends to agree to catch-ups that don't involve dinner, drinks or a movie. Suggest a game of tennis, football, volleyball or hiking in the countryside.
- Have you ever taken a dance class? It's not just a good way to get active, but helps with coordination and can even challenge you mentally.

FIRING UP THE MITOCHONDRIA

Mitochondria are the components of our muscles that act like the combustion chambers in a car engine's cylinders. They take oxygen and fuel – in the case of humans, carbohydrates and fats stored as glycogen in our muscles and liver, and fat deposited as triglycerides in our adipocytes (fat cells) – and combine them to produce the energy that is used to power the movement of contractions in working muscles and keeps us moving.

Increase the pace of your movement and you increase the burning of oxygen and fat within the mitochondria. To keep up, both your heart and lungs have to work harder and faster to deliver calories and oxygen to the hungry muscles.

Train regularly and both the number and activity of the mitochondria in our muscles rise. What that means, in simple terms, is that even when you're not exercising this greater number of active mitochondria will be burning much more energy. This is especially helpful when you are trying to lose stubborn weight and reduce excess fat.

There are many direct benefits specific to aerobic exercise such as calorie burning for weight management, and improved fitness and ability to handle daily activities without losing your breath. Additionally, regular moderate to vigorous aerobic activity can improve your heart health through beneficial changes to cholesterol, triglycerides, blood pressure and inflammation; help control blood sugar, which is good for your metabolism and diabetic risk; increase insulin sensitivity that is essential for reducing cancer risk while activating multiple anti-ageing pathways; boost the production of a hormone called brain-derived neurotrophic factor (BNDF) that exerts powerful protective effects against dementia and depression; and maximise blood and lymph flow which is good for the whole body – especially blood-rich organs like the heart, lungs, brain, kidneys, liver and spleen.

Regular aerobic activity is so important for living a longer healthier life.

BURNING CALORIES: TAKE A CUE FROM VO$_2$

VO$_2$ max is the measurement of oxygen that a person can use during intense exercise. Take, for example, a trained athlete with a VO$_2$ max of 5 litres per minute – they will burn about 1100 calories during an hour-long moderate to intense workout. A sedentary person will likely have a far lower VO$_2$ max. If it's 1.6 litres a minute, they will only burn 360 calories in the same time.

For those of you who have perhaps neglected your exercise routine, it is possible to dramatically improve your VO$_2$ levels quite quickly. After three months of moderate to intense exercise it will typically increase by between 15 and 25 per cent; after two years of exercise it can improve by as much as 50 per cent, depending on how fit you were when you started.

Even just a couple of weeks of exercise can make improvements. Studies show that just five to 10 days of regular aerobic exercising can double aerobic mitochondrial enzymes.

Thinking this just applies to young people, or at least people younger than yourself? Not true. Experiments have shown that even elderly men and women who begin moderate aerobic training can see, within nine months, a 20 per cent increase in muscle mitochondria and therefore calorie consumption.

Anyone who adds regular aerobic exercise to their routine will greatly improve their body's capacity to burn calories.

Consider this: each kilogram of fat contains about 7000 calories. If you're a sedentary person like the one you read about a couple of paragraphs back – the one with a VO$_2$ max of 1.6 litres a minute and only burning 360 calories for every hour of exercise – it'll take about 20 days if you exercise an hour a day to work off that kilo of fat. Improve your VO$_2$ max levels by 20 per cent – as I mentioned before that can take as little as three months – and you'll burn that kilo of fat in 16 days.

Plus, because of increased levels of fitness, you'll actually feel more comfortable exercising for longer because there'll be a lower chance of accumulating lactic acid. That's the stuff that makes you breathe harder, get sore muscles and feel nauseous during strenuous exercise. Aerobic fitness is like investing cash in the bank: the longer you keep at it, the faster it grows.

AEROBIC FITNESS FIGHTS DISEASE

While fitness is great, what we're just as interested in is longevity and staving off chronic illness. Here's how aerobic exercise can help a range of diseases.

CARDIOVASCULAR HEALTH
As well as having positive effects on blood glucose and insulin levels, aerobic exercise when combined with weight loss also increases levels of good cholesterol (HDL-cholesterol) and reduces triglyceride levels and LDL-cholesterol (the bad kind). It also lowers blood pressure and is especially useful for people with hypertension. Aerobic exercise decreases body weight and inflammation, and increases arterial function. All that adds up to a lower chance of suffering from a heart attack or stroke and vascular dementia.

TYPE 2 DIABETES Even in people who are not obese, regular aerobic activity improves insulin sensitivity and glucose tolerance. Studies have shown that more than 56 per cent of diabetic patients who began exercising five to six times a week were able to come off their glucose-lowering medication (compared to just 14.7 per cent of a sedentary control group).

CANCER Studies show that regular aerobic training is associated with a reduced risk of developing at least 13 different types of cancer, particularly breast, colon and endometrial. Endurance exercise reduces abdominal fat, inflammatory cytokines, insulin levels, and IGFI and sex hormones bioavailability, all factors that promote tumour development and growth.

MEMORY PROTECTION The structure of the brain typically deteriorates as we age. Exercise, however, has been linked to profound effects on brain health, helping to protect memory, enhancing attention and thinking skills, and improving the ability to process information. In the short term, it also helps to reduce levels of anxiety and stress, improve mood and self-esteem, and reduce the symptoms of depression. A protein called cathepsin B, whose muscle production is increased during exercise, powerfully increases the circulating level of BDNF. This growth factor promotes the survival of nerve cells and it is as effective at protecting against depression as some antidepressant drugs, but has none of the side effects. Win win.

HARDER, FASTER, STRONGER? EXERCISE TIME REDUCED

The good news, especially if you're someone who has always said you don't have enough time for exercise, is you can exchange longer sessions at a low to medium intensity for shorter sessions at a higher intensity – of which you need at least 75–150 minutes each week, if you decide to take this option.

If you've never come across high-intensity interval training (HIIT) before, it requires working as hard as you can for short bursts, then slowing right down between each interval. So you're gently increasing your heart and breathing rate for a certain amount of time then letting them slow down again and doing that in a repeated pattern.

If you're just starting your HITT regimen, it could be jogging or sprinting on an exercise bike for 4 minutes then slowing down (recovering) for 3 minutes and repeating the pattern three or four times.

You can also try sprint interval training – 60 seconds of high-intensity running, cycling or swimming, 4 minutes recovering – as an option. Start by repeating this just four times. building up to five or six repeats as you get fitter. Do the maths and you'll see you can do a full workout in just 30 minutes.

Take HIIT classes at the gym and you might end up working for intervals of 20 seconds on and 40 seconds off, or 30 seconds on and 30 seconds off, doing five or six types of exercises – anything from squats to riding a stationary bike – in a 'circuit'. It could be that you end up doing the circuit five or six times, depending on what else is included in the class.

As with any type of aerobic exercise, it's important to both gently warm up and cool down at the beginning and end of your HIIT session to avoid injury.

It's thought this type of exercise is equal to or more beneficial for improving cardiovascular health than longer bouts of medium-intensity exercise. It's also helpful for losing weight as it increases the body's metabolism for 24 hours after the session (excess post-exercise oxygen consumption or afterburn effect).

If you're looking for an organic way to add some HIIT to your day, head to the stairs whenever you have a small window of time (perhaps before work, during a coffee break and at lunch time). One small study showed that fitness improved by 12 per cent in sedentary volunteers who vigorously climbed stairs for just 20 seconds three times a day for six weeks.

FITNESS

Fitness we can define as the capacity to do work, or, technically speaking, how well you can get oxygenated blood to working muscles to keep on moving. The fitter you become, the greater your capacity to burn fuel while exercising, with all the benefits of increased blood flow and a metabolism that enables you to burn stored fat more effectively.

HOW FIT ARE YOU?

In exercise science, an athlete's fitness is tracked using the VO_2 max test, which measures the maximum amount of oxygen consumed when we exercise hard (see page 143). You can certainly get this tested, in a specialised health clinic for example, using standardised tests on a treadmill or bicycle.

But an easy (though less precise) way to test yourself at home is by doing the same exercise at the same level, and comparing how you *feel* doing it. For instance, if you have steps and a watch or phone timer, you can pace yourself stepping up and down for 3 minutes at a regular pace, and then rate how breathless you feel right at the end of the 3 minutes and again 3 minutes later. Take note on a scale from 1 to 10 (see opposite), then repeat that exact same test a few weeks later while continuing your aerobic training schedule. When you get fitter your heart and lungs and vessels work better to deliver oxygen and nutrients to your leg muscles, so after a few weeks of training, this exercise should feel easier. You can do this with any aerobic activity, for instance pedalling at 60 rpm for 3 minutes on a stationary bicycle at a set resistance, or swimming laps.

TRACK YOUR FITNESS

So how will you know you are getting fitter?

Perform your own fitness tests every four to six weeks, completing the same activity each time. For instance stepping for 3 minutes at a regular pace, climbing the stairs or on an exercise bike at the same speed and resistance level. At the 3-minute mark, and then again after 3 minutes of sitting rest, note down in your fitness diary your level of perceived exertion (and intensity) and your heart rate.

KNOWING YOUR LEVEL OF PERCEIVED EXERTION (AND INTENSITY):

1 VERY LIGHT hardly moving (like watching TV).

2–3 LIGHT easy to breathe and converse (like a leisurely walk with friends).

4–6 MODERATE becoming noticeably more challenging, breathing hard but can hold a short conversation (like a brisk walk).

7–8 VIGOROUS getting uncomfortable, short of breath and able to speak a sentence (like jogging or running).

9 VERY HARD can barely breathe and speak only a few words (like jogging up a long hill).

10 MAXIMUM EFFORT feels almost impossible to keep going. Completely out of breath and can't talk (like cycling at maximum speed on an exercise bike).

Also record your heart rate (in beats per minute) if you have a device that measures this, or you can measure your heart rate yourself by counting your pulse at your wrist for 15 seconds and multiply by 4 (to get beats per minute).

A WORD ON FITNESS DEVICES

If you are into measuring your fitness, there are a number of tracker devices and wearables which can be excellent when used properly. For instance, a device that accurately measures your heart rate while exercising can tell you whether your heart rate required for the same exercise has changed over a few weeks – the fitter you become, the lower your resting heart rate, as well as the heart rate you need during a given activity like the step test mentioned opposite.

Devices that record footsteps might tell you the total volume of exercise you do, but not the intensity of exercise or your body's fitness.

CAN YOU DO MORE ONE DAY TO MAKE UP FOR THE REST OF THE WEEK?

If you decide to do a five-hour hike on a Sunday, that's great, but it won't make up for being sedentary the rest of the week.

Your aim is daily blocks of at least 30 minutes, exercise with lots of 2–5 minute movement breaks scattered throughout each day. Even two hours of uninterrupted sitting starts to wreak havoc with your metabolism. This is why being laid up in hospital is so unpleasant, and also why we've changed post-surgical physical rehabilitation to try to get people mobile and walking as soon as practicable afterwards, where once we just encouraged complete bed rest.

WHAT TIME OF DAY IS BEST?

The answer is the time you will stick to a new habit of course! Some find exercising before breakfast is easiest to fit in their day, and there is evidence you will burn off more fat by doing your aerobic activity on an empty stomach. However, find a time that works for you and commit to it. Block it out in your diary. Maybe even coordinate with a friend or family member to join you – accountability together helps.

WHAT IF I CAN'T FIT 30 MINUTES IN EVERY DAY?

There are a few options for you to build up aerobic fitness if, like many of us, you might not have up to 60 minutes a day in a block for exercise.

Set a timer so that every 30 minutes to 1 hour you are reminded to stand and move around: take 30 steps, do some stretches or some resistance exercises like push-ups or squats. This is especially useful if you are in a job that involves a lot of sitting. Long uninterrupted sitting time can lead to increased risks of heart disease and type 2 diabetes – not to mention you just feel sluggish and lethargic after a while. By doing 3–4 minutes of activity every hour you can accumulate the minimum 30 minutes of activity for the day.

> 3–4 minutes of activity every hour quickly adds up to 30 minutes a day!

FITNESS AND INTERVAL TRAINING

Interval training is where you alternate low and either high-, or moderate-intensity exercise. This is a very well-researched format for getting the cardiovascular and metabolic benefits of all that long-distance exercise in a shorter period of time. Sounds great right? Just be aware of two caveats when doing interval training:

- Caveat 1 – You have to be able to perform moderate–high intensity exercise safely. This includes having both the strength to handle high intensity, as well as the right place and equipment.

- Caveat 2 – You won't burn off as many overall calories for the same cardiovascular and metabolic benefit as doing low–moderate exercise for long periods.

If you're just starting a new exercise program, it is better to wait until you've built up a good baseline of fitness and strength before attempting higher intensities with your aerobic exercise. This is especially true of things like running, where a good rule of thumb is to only start a HIIT program when you can comfortably jog for at least 20 minutes continuously.

Cycling is a much safer aerobic exercise due to its low impact, and studies on HIIT are most often done with indoor cycle machines, so you may be able to start HIIT sooner if you've got access to a spin or exercise bike. Remember start low and go slow before you sprint.

If you've got the ability and the place though, moderate intensity interval training (MIIT) and high-intensity interval training (HIIT) are excellent ways to gain the fitness and metabolic benefits of aerobic exercise, fast!

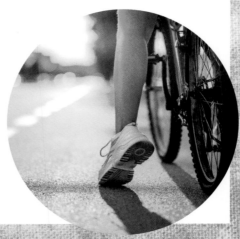

How do you perform MIIT and HIIT?

- *Frequency* – perform MIIT/HIIT up to three times a week, as your aerobic training. More than this and you might wear yourself out, as it is quite demanding on muscles and joints.
- *Intensity*
  - for MIIT: take yourself up to an intensity of 6–7.5 to 10 during the intervals.
  - for HIIT: take yourself up to an intensity of 8–9 to 10 or, if you are well-trained already and performing a safe activity like a stationary cycle, treadmill, or a level running track – 9–10 to 10.
- *Time* – per session, MIIT up to 60 minutes total, and HIIT up to 30 minutes. This *includes* warm up and cool down, which you definitely do not want to skip, given your muscles will be working hard.
- *Type* – any safe aerobic exercise you have some skill at already like cycling, running, rowing, swimming, and that enables you to reach the necessary intensity.
- *Volume*
  - for MIIT: up to 180 minutes a week (counts to your moderate intensity target of 150–300 minutes a week).
  - for HIIT: up to 90 minutes a week (counts to your vigorous intensity target of 75–150 minutes a week).
- *Progression* – intensity is your guide to progressing interval training, as you want to hit your intensity targets for each interval.

Lift your intensity with MIIT or HIIT and reduce the time you spend on strength training.

INTENSITY

The intensity of a physical activity is how hard you feel you are working while doing it. The more intense an activity, the harder it feels to do, the more oxygen, calories, and fuel you require to complete it. However, your level of fatigue can build up quickly the harder the heart, lungs, and even brain have to work to keep up. You'll feel this as muscles burning, increased breathing, higher heart rate and fatigue.

The less intense an activity, the longer you can do it without getting too tired. You will notice an increase in breathing and heart rate, but you are unlikely to get sore muscles unless you are moving for a long time.

To start with, most of your exercise time of 150–300 minutes a week should be spent at a low to moderate intensity, with higher intensity exercise when you have built up a good base of fitness and strength.

Moderate intensity includes some of the most fun and engaging forms of exercise once you've built up to it. Most aerobic and dance classes are pitched at a moderate intensity, including step ups, light jogging, movement patterns that get your brain working as well as your body, and often resistance, balance, and flexibility thrown in to boot. Playing tennis, football and volleyball and dancing classes are not only fun, but a great way to socialise and train those parts of your brain responsible for learning new motor skills. Win win!

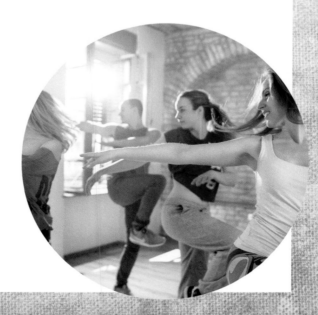

WHY DO WE WANT INTENSITY?

Higher intensities create more change, faster. This change can mean getting fitter, feeling less out of breath in your other activities, having more energy, getting stronger, feeling generally more able. On the inside, these changes are reflected in greater fat burning ability, change in body composition (more muscle, less fat, stronger bones) and improved insulin sensitivity. Your body adapts to higher intensity by making all these changes – for the simple intention of making that same activity *less* intense next time!

This is the secret to feeling healthy and able through your lifespan: spending some time challenging your body with higher intensity activity actually gives you a physiological and psychological reserve capacity for everything else you do in your life.

There's two ways we use intensity in our training program:

1. to record how hard you feel you're exercising now; and
2. to use this to progress your exercise next time, so you maintain the right intensity.

Here's an example.

Let's say you started out being able to only walk 1 kilometre (half a mile) on flat ground in 15 minutes before having to stop and catch your breath. During the walk you felt like you were at an intensity of 7, and at the end of that walk, you might feel you reached an intensity of 8.

If you kept walking this same 1 kilometre (half a mile) a few times over the next month, you'd gradually feel it was less effort. You'd be able to walk the same distance faster or be able to walk further in 15 minutes, before running out of breath. Your intensity might drop to 6 or even 5. It's become much easier.

All those adaptations your body made in response to your 7–8 walking – increased strength and fitness, better fat burning ability, better coordination – start to drop off a little when it only feels 5–6. So in order to keep gaining those same benefits, you'd have to get back up to a 7–8 for that walk.

HOW CAN YOU INCREASE THE INTENSITY OF AN ACTIVITY?

For aerobic exercise, you can increase intensity by:

- moving faster – jogging rather than walking
- increasing distance
- exercising for a longer time
- using harder variations – walking up hills or stairs, rather than on the flat
- increasing the resistance on the exercise – changing the amount of drag on the gears for a stationary exercise bike, or elliptical trainer; or carrying hand weights/ankle weights on a walk.

INTENSITY TARGETS

You want to spend most of your 150–300 minutes a week of exercise at a moderate intensity between 3–6; and alternatively, for those who can perform the activity safely, up to 75 minutes a week of vigorous intensity, between 7–9. Reserve 10 for high-intensity interval training, only when you have had at least three months of regular aerobic training.

- Use the scale (page 147) to record your own intensity, by asking yourself the question: *At what intensity out of 10 am I working at the moment?*

- Use this to help reach your intensity goals – by increasing the intensity of your exercises over time so you stay in a range that continues to help your body adapt and get fitter, stronger, and feel more able.

KEEP A DIARY

You can use a fitness diary, a fitness tracker and app, or a typed journal to record each day of your fitness calendar:

- time spent exercising (don't forget to add in bite-size exercise breaks during your day)
- details of what you did – i.e. 30 minutes: jogged every 3 minutes for 1 minute and walked the rest; or with a fitness tracker, you might record the distance you covered cycling or swimming
- intensity of your session e.g. 4 for walking, 6–8 for jogging.

In order to gain the most benefits you need to step up the intensity!

TYPE OF EXERCISE: LOW, MODERATE, HIGH IMPACT

There are lots of types of aerobic activity to spread through your exercise week. Let's split them up into low, moderate and high impact. Low impact is, as the name suggests, easier on joints and spine. This is a good choice when you have pain in places like your knees, hip, or lower back, or are less steady on your feet than you would like. High impact will require you to be relatively pain free before engaging in that exercise type, and safely able to perform it.

LOW-IMPACT ACTIVITIES

Walk, swim, bicycle (outdoors or stationary), elliptical training machine, rowing (outdoors on the water or indoors on a rowing machine), hand crank machine, ski ergometer machine.

Choose the majority of your 150–300 minutes from this type. Start slow and build up your pace and intensity over time; it is better to have a good base of getting your body used to exercise when starting a new program. This allows time for your joints and muscles to strengthen.

Just remember you will need to challenge yourself. Your body naturally wants to make all movement more efficient and adapts to an exercise so that after a few weeks of the same thing, you'll end up burning fewer calories. Track how fast you are walking, cycling, running or swimming – whichever aerobic exercise you choose – then build in extra speed or difficulty every three or four weeks or so to maintain yourself at the right intensity.

MODERATE-IMPACT ACTIVITIES

Moderate-impact exercise like jogging, stair climbing (outside, indoors, or machine), dancing or aerobics classes mean you will strike the ground harder than when you, say, go for a walk. There are many benefits to having this impact, notably on bone health. The vibration caused by impact, plus your body weight landing on the ground from a short distance, as in jogging or stair climbing, gives your bones hundreds of little stimuli to break down a little, and a stimulus to repair stronger. This is why moderate impact is recommended for those at risk of developing osteoporosis.

HIGH-IMPACT ACTIVITIES

High-impact exercise is where you'll spend very little time in your usual training program, unless you are an advanced exerciser, athlete or into competitive sports and you have built up good experience and coordination. This includes long-distance running, sprinting, obstacle courses, jumping and also sports like football, rugby, boxing, hockey, skiing, tennis, squash, basketball, volleyball, and netball.

There are stronger benefits for bone density than low or moderate impact, but you're also more likely to gain an injury which could have worse long-term outcomes for bone and joint health. That said, a lot of people who are conditioned to running, jumping, and contact with either balls or other players, do have a lot of fun and satisfaction from things like competitive sports or a fast run. For the advanced exerciser, high impact like running long distance may be their primary choice of weekly activity.

When you're building up fitness, and certainly if you are wishing to minimise risk of injury and falling if you are a little unsteady on your feet, high-impact activities can be more problematic than beneficial. For those conditioned to them, like sportspeople and athletes, the risks of injury are reduced because of adaptations in muscles, joints, and, most importantly, how their brain coordinates and controls movement.

A WARNING FOR THOSE WITH EXISTING PROBLEMS

For those with sore and misaligned joints, instability on their feet, or existing bone disease, moderate intensity like jogging might be too strong. In this case, see a physiotherapist and start with low impact and build up strength and stability before attempting moderate intensity. You want to be exercising safely and effectively for life – there's no point in getting an injury that puts you out of action!

If you are experiencing joint pain, arthritis, or other conditions that might make you unsteady on your feet, another great help is strength training (see page 158), as this can be done safely, with less impact, but helps remodel muscles, bones and joints as well.

AEROBIC EXERCISE PLAN

Now that we've covered the basics of aerobic exercise, let's put together a three-stage fitness program: initial conditioning, improvement and maintenance.

INITIAL CONDITIONING

For most people who haven't been exercising, it normally takes between four to six weeks to gain a level of conditioning once they start exercising regularly. During this initial stage you are likely to experience the greatest fitness improvements. (Already fit men and women can skip this stage altogether and move directly to the Improvement stage.)

The best exercising choices for this initial stage are low to medium intensity aerobic activities in conjunction with stretch exercises.

When you start out, you should begin exercising for 15 to 20 minutes on alternate days, increasing to 30 minutes over a four to six week period.

IMPROVEMENT STAGE

This stage should last between four to five months as you gradually build your conditioning and undertake more intense, longer and more frequent exercise sessions. You should increase how long you exercise for every two to three weeks, and increase the frequency of exercising from three to five times a week. It's important to remember that the intensity, duration and frequency should never be increased together.

MAINTENANCE STAGE

It usually takes about six months to reach this stage. Once you have achieved a reasonable level of fitness you can undertake a mixture of moderately hard aerobic workouts and activities you enjoy like soccer, volleyball, basketball with friends, dancing etc. It's a great idea to vary your activities so that it remains enjoyable and fun. For example if you were riding a bike five days a week at the end of the improvement stage, you could change that to only three times a week and play tennis or swim on the other two days.

Perform aerobic exercise once you have reached the Maintenance stage, at least 30 minutes a day and up to 60 minutes (150–300 minutes a week). Use a variety of aerobic exercises that you are confident you can do, and that you enjoy, such as walking, swimming, jogging, cycling, rowing, dancing, cross-country skiing, aerobics classes, etc. Consider high-impact exercise when you have built up good strength, joint health and confidence.

Use the scale (page 147) to gauge how hard you are working – ask yourself while you are exercising: *At what intensity out of 10 am I working at the moment?*

- 4–6 out of 10 is *moderate*, and that's a level you can use for your full 150–300 minutes per week, OR

- 7–9 is *vigorous*, and if you can do this safely, you can do 75–150 minutes per week at this level rather than the full 150–300 minutes.

- Only go to 10 if you are confident you can be safe, and have good experience with your chosen exercise, e.g. stationary cycling or rowing.

- You can use HIIT, where you alternate between moderate and safe vigorous intensity in one session, to count as *vigorous* exercise, so saving time in your week.

- Keep your intensity levels up by deliberately progressing your exercise by going faster, further, or harder, as you get fitter and more able.

- If you can, exercise with friends, in a group, or in classes led by trained fitness instructors, to help you gain extra motivation, accountability and guidance.

- Use bite-size exercise breaks of 3–5 minutes every hour or so, while working or sitting for long periods. Go for a quick walk, jog on the spot, do some squats or push-ups – you'll add to your daily time spent exercising as well as boost your metabolism and brain function at the same time.

- Plan and track your aerobic exercise *daily* and *weekly*, so you can see improvements and feel engaged in your progress – this is key to long-term habit formation!

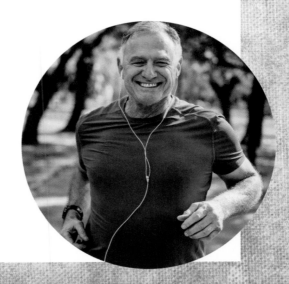

STRENGTH TRAINING

Of course, strength is very important to everyday life. We need it to climb stairs, carry our shopping, lift a bag overhead, pick up our children and grandchildren, even open a jar. Not just that, but muscle mass and strength is also important for bone health. Live a sedentary life and you're at risk of losing so much muscle mass and strength that you end up becoming frail and dependent on others for simple activities, like dressing or getting out of bed. Plus, take a fall – more possible if you become frail – and you could end up breaking bones and becoming bedridden.

Even if you have been sedentary for many years, there is good news because including more physical activity in your life, especially muscle-strengthening exercise, can quickly counteract loss of muscle and bone mass, and progressively rebuild strength.

Added to those benefits, strength training can help with weight loss because it increases our resting metabolic rate even after we stop exercising (a biological phenomenon called excess post-exercise oxygen consumption).

Strength, in addition to cardiorespiratory fitness, is something that blesses our bodies with youthful ability and stamina, but is something we tend to lose with disuse. It is related to the amount of muscle mass you have and how well you can drive this muscle with your brain – what we would call neuromuscular strength. Muscle is also very metabolically active, much more so than stored fat, so there's a potential huge benefit to maintaining or adding muscle with strength-building exercises, the second major part of this exercise plan.

Strength is something we tend to overlook until it becomes a problem – like if you've ever tried to walk after a period of illness or immobility, and find your legs are almost too weak to hold you up. We gradually lose muscle mass and strength as we age too, but this happens over decades.

The wonderful thing is we can build muscle mass, strength and resilience at any age, and the benefits are *enormous*. Muscle strengthening activities can help you feel better by directly impacting mood and mental health; can help you reshape your body so you move, function and look better; build bone strength; and burn more calories, so help with weight management.

BUILDING STRENGTH - HOW DOES IT WORK?

The principle of building strength and metabolically healthy muscles is movement against a resistance to cause fatigue and microscopic damage or tears to the muscle cells, followed by activation of stem cells and repair.

1. Perform a movement (pull, push, squat, lunge, bend, twist);

2. Against some sort of resistance (your own body weight; an elastic exercise band; a weight such as a dumbbell, a bag, or even items lying around your home; or an exercise machine);

3. To fatigue – i.e. you can't successfully perform that movement again because your muscles have run out of energy;

4. Allow the muscles to recover for enough time to complete the exercise again.

When you repeat this process, your muscles, bones and joints adapt to all that additional work by getting stronger, toned, sometimes bigger, and definitely more metabolically active.

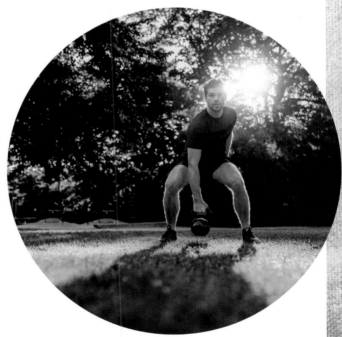

HOW IT FITS INTO YOUR PROGRAM

When people think of muscle-strengthening exercises they tend to think of barbells, weights and bodybuilding, but it is far less complicated than that. You can use your own body weight to perform any number of strengthening exercises. Add some small weights and resistance bands and you can easily perform strength workouts in your own home.

You need to do at least two strength training workouts per week, from 20 minutes to 60 minutes each, covering all the major muscle groups. This includes abdominals and middle and lower back (core), the chest, shoulders, arms, hips and thighs. Each week we should aim to build strength, and larger, better functioning muscles, to help us thrive mentally and metabolically for a healthy longevity.

How strength training differs from aerobic training is in the activities we do, and the resistance used. Rather than a rhythmic movement done over many minutes, like walking or cycling, strength exercises involve working against some form of resistance, like a weight, an elastic band, or machine, so that your muscles fatigue after 6 to 15 repetitions. It is this fatigue that stimulates our muscles to regrow stronger, and as a result help our metabolism, when we recover in between workouts.

Don't be too concerned about gaining muscle mass and becoming 'bulky' as a result. It takes a lot of effort and many hours to start to gain a bodybuilder physique. For longevity we just want well-functioning, metabolically active muscles that enable us to move well and feel good doing so!

DO I HAVE TO DO TWO LONG SESSIONS?

The main thing about building strong, metabolically active muscles is regular activity that challenges them beyond just everyday movements. You can do the same amount of time but split into three 30-minute sessions or four 20-minute sessions. You can even add additional sessions, if you want to reshape your body and add more muscle mass or help strengthen your bones, for example. However, the minimum to achieve all the benefits of building strength is exercising each major muscle group until they reach a good level of fatigue, twice a week.

STRUCTURING THE WORKOUT – SETS AND REPS AND REST

Each of your strength workouts should include around 8 to 10 different exercises covering the whole body. For each of these exercises, you'll do a certain number of repetitions (reps) to try and reach muscular fatigue (which creates our get-strong and build-healthy-muscle signals). After one set of repetitions, you rest for a brief period, before repeating the set.

For instance, three sets of eight repetitions of a squat would mean:

Squat 8 times, then rest 60 seconds.

Squat another 8 times, then rest 60 seconds.

Squat 8 times again, then move on to the next exercise, like a wall push-up.

So, all up your strength workouts will be twice a week 8–10 exercises, and each will comprise two to three sets of 6 to 15 repetitions – aiming for about 45 minutes each session.

HOW TO APPROACH STRENGTH TRAINING IF YOU'RE NEW TO IT

One of the things people starting strength training need to think about is just practising each new movement. Like dancing, or learning to drive a car, it feels awkward at first as the muscles and joints have to learn to move together to do the work. You also want to think about developing these as lifelong movement skills that can become almost automatic – like driving a car – so they feel comfortable, and you feel confident doing them.

For example with squats, your first few weeks should just be about practising the movement. Go into the workout with the mindset that you want to get better at the *movement*, and only then when you've built up some confidence in the movement, you add resistance like a weight or band.

> This is not about becoming a body builder – this will build your strength enabling you to move well.

INTENSITY FOR STRENGTH EXERCISE

Gauging intensity with strength exercise is a bit different to aerobic activity – but not by much.

While performing the exercise you still want to ask yourself: *At what intensity do I feel I am exercising?* But also you need to ask yourself: *How many more repetitions could I manage at this resistance level?*

Whenever you're doing weight training exercise – and that includes when you're performing moves that use your own body weight – it's important to breathe in, during the easy part of the movement and exhale as you 'lift' to prevent a dangerous rise in blood pressure. Need an example? During a squat, breathe in as you bend your knees and lower yourself then exhale as you return to standing upright. If you're doing a push-up, breathe in as you lower yourself towards the floor and exhale as you push away and straighten your arms again.

Always perform strength exercises in a slow and controlled fashion. Ensure you retain good posture at all times, and engage your core. What does that mean? Tightening and bracing the muscles of your core – the abdominals, hip flexors, glutes and any others that make up your muscle 'corset' – to keep your spine safe and stable.

Maintaining form, as you'll hear the experts say, protects you from injury to your muscles, spine and joints. It will also help you get the most from every movement.

You also need to rest for 48 hours between strength sessions to ensure your muscles can recover, grow and strengthen.

> To build strong metabolically healthy muscles you need to challenge them regularly beyond just everyday movement.

STRENGTH TRAINING PROGRAM

MUSCLE GROUP	BEGINNER FIRST 8 WEEKS 12–15 REPS, 2–3 SETS EACH	INTERMEDIATE LEVEL 1 – SECOND 8 WEEKS 10–12 REPS, 2–3 SETS EACH	INTERMEDIATE LEVEL 2 – THIRD 8 WEEKS 8–10 REPS, 2–3 SETS EACH
THIGHS (QUADRICEPS)	Squats onto bench	Squat to stand on one leg	Step backs
CHEST	Wall or bench push ups	Push ups from knees	Push ups
THIGHS (HAMSTRINGS)	Toe touches	Deadlift	Wide stance deadlift
UPPER BACK	Band pulls – two handed	Band pulls	Band pulls – one hand
HIPS AND LOWER BACK	Glute bridge	Feet together/feet-wide glute bridge	Glute bridge single
SHOULDERS (DELTOIDS)	Front raise	Single arm overhead press	Two-hand overhead press
HIPS SUPPORT	Single leg bendovers with support	Single leg bendover	Side hops
SHOULDER SUPPORT	Wall external rotations	Band pull-apart	Butterflies
CORE AND ABDOMINALS	McGill crunch	Plank from knees Plank from toes	Leg scissors
ARMS (BICEPS)	Bicep curl	Band bicep curl	Band bicep curl
ARMS (TRICEPS)	Isometric dip	Isometric dip	Dips

STRENGTH TRAINING EXERCISES
BEGINNERS
REPS 12–15 × 2–3 SETS
FIRST 8 WEEKS

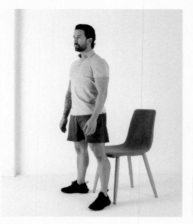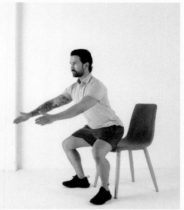

THIGHS (QUADRICEPS): Squats onto bench
Standing with your feet shoulder-width apart
(about 30 cm / 1 ft) in front of a sturdy chair, bench,
or couch, slowly lower your hips toward the bench
as if you are going to sit down. Rather than putting
your weight on the bench, pause for a moment
then squeeze your buttocks and smoothly stand
up straight again. The lower the bench, the harder
this becomes.

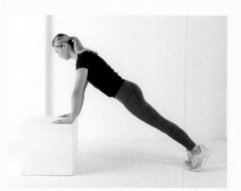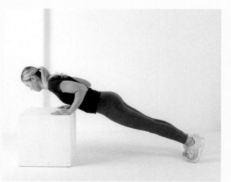

CHEST: Bench push ups
Starting with arms outstretched and back straight,
slowly lower yourself towards a solid surface like a
bench, table, or wall. Using your arms and shoulders
push back up to the starting position.

BEGINNERS
REPS 12–15 × 2–3 SETS
FIRST 8 WEEKS

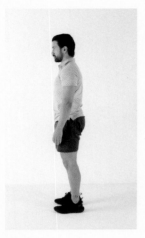
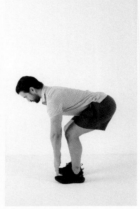

THIGHS (HAMSTRINGS):
Toe touches
Without weights, or light band/ weights only. Stand tall, feet shoulder-width apart, hands on the front of your thighs. Keeping your spine straight, start by hingeing at your hips, and bending your knees. Lower your hands towards your toes until you feel a little stretch at the back of your legs. Pause for a second, then breathe out and return to standing up straight. Be mindful to not remain bent over, or straighten up too quickly if you have low blood pressure or get dizzy when standing up quickly.

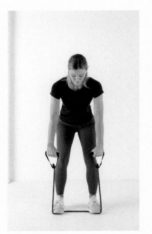
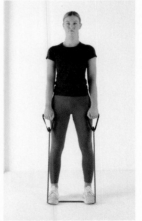

UPPER BACK: Band pulls two handed
With a secure anchor for your band and knees bent, stand tall with feet apart, and pull both hands in toward the side of your body. Keep your chest up, no slouching! Slowly return to knees bent and arms fully extended, and repeat the pull.

BEGINNERS
REPS 12–15 × 2–3 SETS
FIRST 8 WEEKS

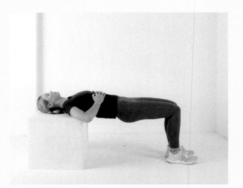
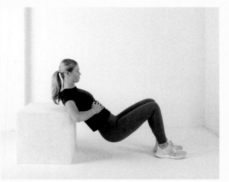

HIPS AND LOWER BACK: Glute bridge
Start with your upper back resting on the edge of a cushioned bench, sturdy chair or couch, body and thighs parallel to the ground, feet shoulder-width apart. Slowly lower your hips. Hold briefly, then squeeze through your buttocks back to the start position.

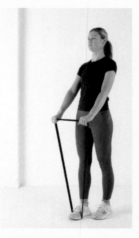
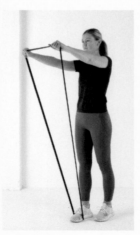

SHOULDERS (DELTOIDS): Front raise
With either bands or weights. Stand tall with feet apart and chest out, arms straight. Lift both arms forward, to shoulder height, then slowly return to the start position.

BEGINNERS
REPS 12–15 × 2–3 SETS
FIRST 8 WEEKS

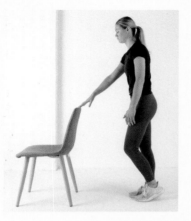
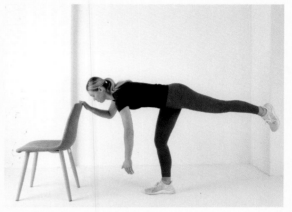

HIPS SUPPORT: Single leg bendovers with support
Keeping your left hand on something solid for
support, slowly lower your left hand towards your
right toe while extending your left leg backwards.
Complete all reps on one side, then change sides.

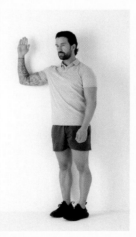
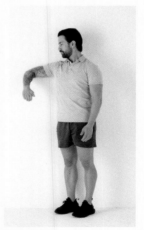

SHOULDER SUPPORT: Wall external rotations
With your elbow bent at 90 degrees and upper arm
against a wall at shoulder height, rotate your upper
arm to move the back of your hand towards the wall.
Hold for 3 seconds, lower as far as you can without
lifting your arm off the wall, then repeat.

BEGINNERS
REPS 12–15 × 2–3 SETS
FIRST 8 WEEKS

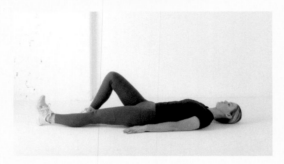

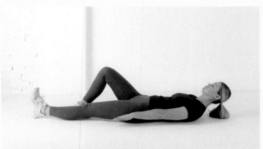

CORE AND ABDOMINALS: McGill crunch
Lie on your back, hands by your sides or under
your lower back. Keep one knee bent. Tighten your
stomach and keeping your lower back from lifting off
the ground or your hands, lift your chest and head
off the ground. This does not have to be far off the
ground to feel it in your abdominal muscles! Hold for
5 seconds then return to the ground. Aim to build up
to 10 second holds repeated 6–8 times per side.

BEGINNERS
REPS 12–15 × 2–3 SETS
FIRST 8 WEEKS

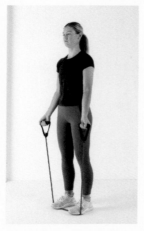 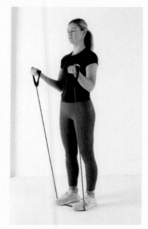

ARMS (BICEPS): Bicep curl
With either bands or weights. Keep elbows beside your body, shoulders back and chest out while you bring your hands to shoulder height, then slowly return to the start position.

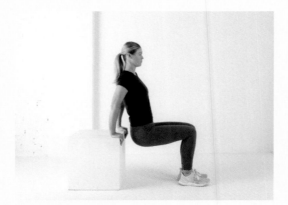

ARMS (TRICEPS): Isometric dip
Sitting on the edge of a sturdy bench, chair, or low wall, place hands beside your hips. Take your weight in your hands. If you feel able, you can support more bodyweight by moving your hips forward off the bench. Hold for 5 seconds, then rest. Build up to 15–20 second holds.

STRENGTH TRAINING EXERCISES
INTERMEDIATE: LEVEL 1
REPS 10–12 × 2–3 SETS
SECOND 8 WEEKS

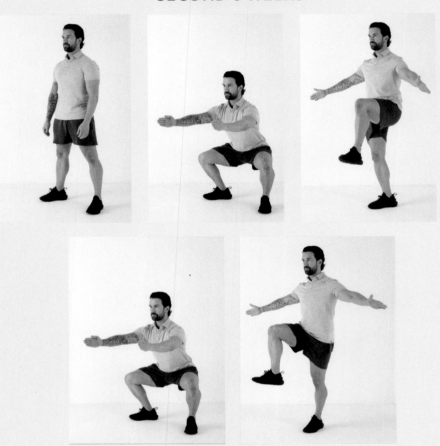

THIGHS (QUADRICEPS): Squat to stand on one leg
Standing with feet shoulder-width apart, slowly lower your hips towards the ground as if you were going to sit down, keeping your chest and chin up. Lower as far as you feel comfortable while keeping your heels on the ground and spine straight. Squeeze your buttocks and smoothly stand up straight again. At the top position, come up onto one foot to balance for at least a second, then step your foot back down into the start position. Repeat by alternating the leg you balance on at the top position. Use this exercise to build up balance. If you struggle to balance on one leg initially, keep working on the Single Leg Bendovers with Support (page 167), or add a support (something solid to hold onto like a chair back) while standing at the top of this exercise on one leg.

INTERMEDIATE: LEVEL 2
REPS 10–12 × 2–3 SETS
THIRD 8 WEEKS

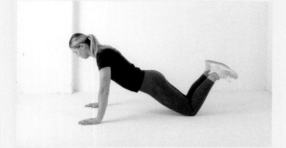
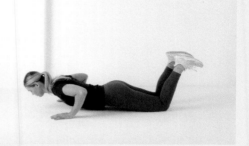

CHEST: Push ups from knees
Starting on your knees with arms outstretched and back straight, slowly lower yourself towards the ground. Push back up to start position through your arms and shoulders.

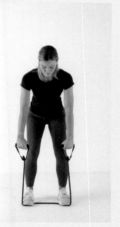
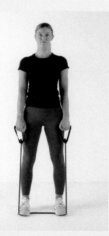
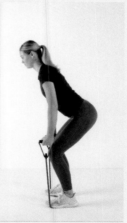
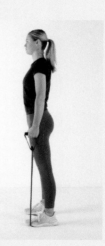

THIGHS (HAMSTRINGS): Deadlift
Use a band or weights. With feet shoulder-width apart, keep your spine straight, and hinging at your hips, lean forward to move your hands towards your feet. Keep your knees over your feet, don't let them cave inward. Squeeze your buttocks to stand back up straight.

INTERMEDIATE: LEVEL 1
REPS 10–12 × 2–3 SETS
SECOND 8 WEEKS

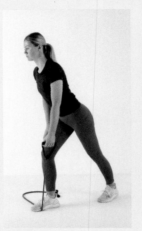 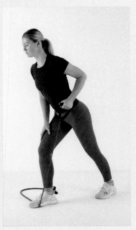

UPPER BACK: Band pulls
With either a dumbbell or band, maintain a straight back while leaning forward at the hips and pull towards the side of your body. Return slowly to a straight arm position.

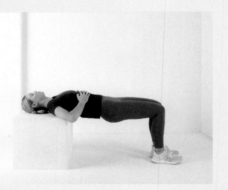 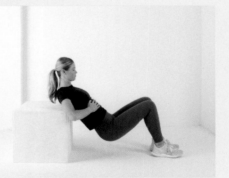

HIPS AND LOWER BACK: Feet together/feet wide glute bridge
Start with your upper back resting on the edge of a cushioned bench, sturdy chair or couch, body and thighs parallel to the ground, feet next to each other. Slowly lower your hips. Hold briefly, then squeeze through your buttocks back to the start position. Repeat with the next set feet wider than shoulder-width apart.

INTERMEDIATE: LEVEL 1
REPS 10–12 × 2–3 SETS
SECOND 8 WEEKS

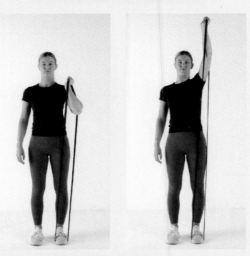

SHOULDERS (DELTOIDS): Single arm overhead press
This is a one-handed version of an overhead press.
It can be done with either a band or a weight (e.g. a
dumbbell). Only do this if you can comfortably raise
your arm above shoulder height, otherwise continue
with the Front Raise (page 166).

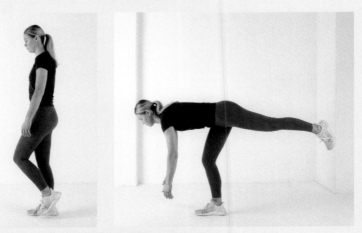

HIPS SUPPORT: Single leg bendover
From standing, slowly lower your left hand towards
your right toe while extending your left leg backwards.
Complete all reps on one side, then change sides.

INTERMEDIATE: LEVEL 1
REPS 10–12 × 2–3 SETS
SECOND 8 WEEKS

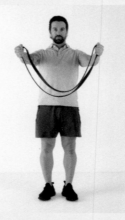 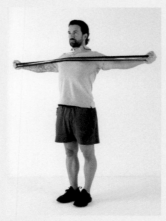

SHOULDER SUPPORT: Band pull-apart
Stand tall with chest out. Pull the band apart until it touches the middle of your chest, pause for 1–2 seconds, and return to rest. You can adjust the difficulty with either a stronger band or shorten the length of the band you use.

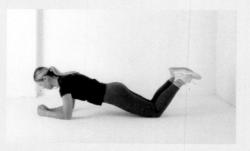 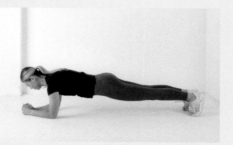

CORE AND ABDOMINALS: Plank from knees
Keep your spine straight and tighten your stomach muscles, hold for 15 seconds. Work your way up to a total of 60 seconds, either all at once, or 4 × 15 seconds with 5 second rests between.

CORE AND ABDOMINALS: Plank from toes
Keep your spine straight and tighten your stomach muscles, hold for 15 seconds. Work your way up to a total of 60 seconds, either all at once, or 4 × 15 seconds with 5 second rests between.

INTERMEDIATE: LEVEL 1
REPS 10–12 × 2–3 SETS
SECOND 8 WEEKS

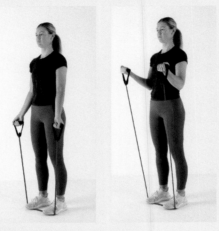

ARMS (BICEPS): Bicep curl
Use either bands or weights. Keep elbows beside your body, shoulders back and chest out while you bring your hands to shoulder height and slowly return.

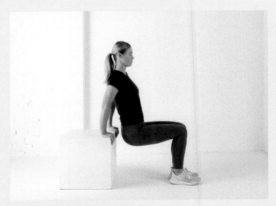

ARMS (TRICEPS): Isometric dip
Sitting on the edge of a sturdy bench, chair or low wall, place hands beside your hips. Take your weight in your hands. If you feel able, you can support more bodyweight by moving your hips forward off the bench. Hold for 5 seconds, then rest. Build up to 15–20 second holds.

STRENGTH TRAINING EXERCISES
INTERMEDIATE: LEVEL 2
REPS 10–12 × 2–3 SETS
THIRD 8 WEEKS

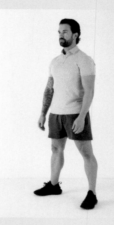
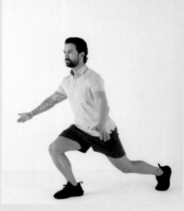

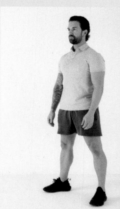
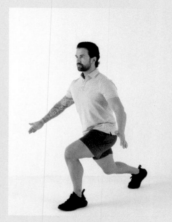
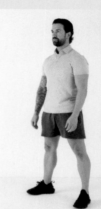

THIGHS (QUADRICEPS): Step backs

Start from a standing position, feet together, lift one foot and place it on the ground a comfortable distance behind you. Staying balanced, slowly bend your forward knee and lower yourself toward the ground. Lower only as far as your knee feels comfortable, then return to start. Alternate legs. An alternative to stepping backward is to step up onto a solid bench or step with one leg, then slowly lower back to the ground supporting yourself on the one leg.

INTERMEDIATE: LEVEL 2
REPS 10–12 × 2–3 SETS
THIRD 8 WEEKS

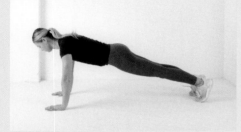

CHEST: Push ups
Starting with arms outstretched and back straight, toes on the ground, slowly lower yourself towards the ground. Push back up to the start position through your arms and shoulders.

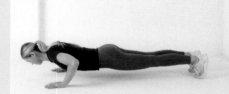

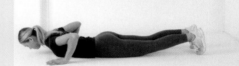

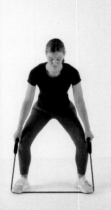
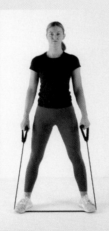
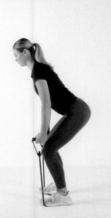
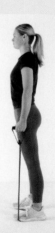

THIGHS (HAMSTRINGS): Wide stance deadlift
Band or weights. With feet twice shoulder-width apart, keep your spine straight, and hinging at your hips, lean forward to move your hands towards your feet. Keep your knees over your feet, don't let them cave inward. Squeeze your buttocks to stand back up straight.

INTERMEDIATE: LEVEL 2
REPS 10–12 × 2–3 SETS
THIRD 8 WEEKS

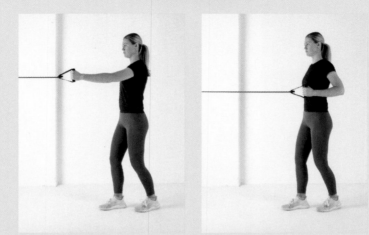

UPPER BACK: Band pulls – one hand
With a secure anchor for your band, pull toward the side of your body with one hand. Slowly return to full stretch.

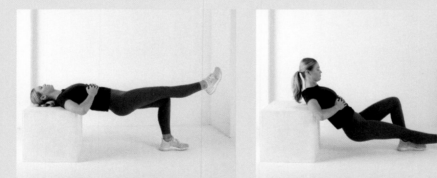

HIPS AND LOWER BACK: Glute bridge single
Start with your upper back resting on the edge of a cushioned bench, sturdy chair or couch, body and thighs parallel to the ground, and one leg extended. Slowly lower your hips. Hold briefly, then squeeze through your buttocks back to the start position. Complete all reps on one leg before changing to the other leg.

INTERMEDIATE: LEVEL 2
REPS 10–12 × 2–3 SETS
THIRD 8 WEEKS

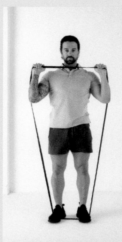 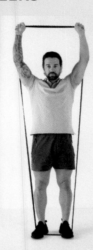

SHOULDERS (DELTOIDS): Two-hand overhead press
This is the two-handed version of an overhead press. It can be done with either a band or a weight (e.g. a dumbbell).Only do this if you can comfortably raise your arm above shoulder height, otherwise continue with the Front Raise (page 166).

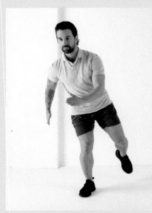 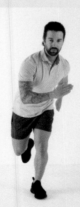

HIPS SUPPORT: Side hops
Start by balancing on one foot. Hop over an imaginary line on the ground to your other foot. As you gain balance and strength, you can increase the width you hop.

INTERMEDIATE: LEVEL 2
REPS 10–12 × 2–3 SETS
THIRD 8 WEEKS

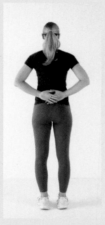
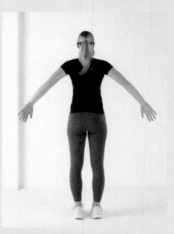
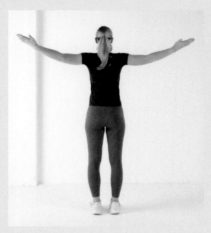

SHOULDER SUPPORT: Butterflies
This can be performed standing, or lying face down on the ground or a mat with your head and chest lifted 2–4 cm. Tuck your hands together behind your lower back. Lift them off your back, then extend both arms below your bottom and sweep them in a big arc out to 90 degrees from your body. Finish with arms outstretched and your thumbs pointing backwards. Return hands to rest behind your lower back for one rep.

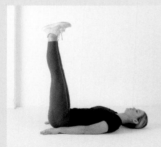
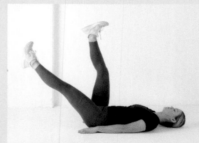
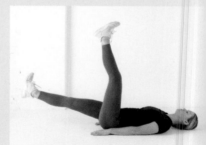

CORE AND ABDOMINALS: Leg scissors
Lying on your back, extend both legs straight into the air. Slowly lower one leg at a time. Only lower them as far as you can still keep your lower back from arching off the ground.

INTERMEDIATE: LEVEL 2
REPS 10–12 × 2–3 SETS
THIRD 8 WEEKS

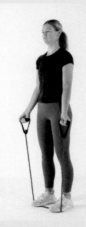 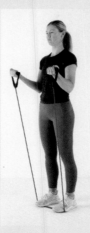

ARMS (BICEPS): Band bicep curl
With either bands or weights. Keep elbows
beside your body, shoulders back and chest
out while you bring your hands to shoulder
height and slowly return.

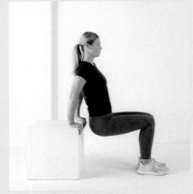 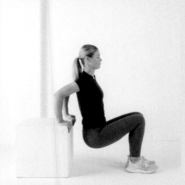

ARMS (TRICEPS): Dips
Sitting on the edge of a sturdy bench, chair, or low wall, place
hands beside your hips. Take your weight in your hands.
Support your bodyweight by moving your hips forward off the
bench, and slowly lower your hips toward the ground. Only go
as far down as you feel comfortable through the shoulder, while
keeping your chest up and out (don't slump!). Push through the
back of the arms back up to start position.

ALL IN BALANCE

Posture, balance and joint flexibility are often overlooked in fitness plans. Ignore them at your peril – the health effects of poor posture, lack of balance, and joint misalignment and stiffness affect many aspects of daily life and contribute to disease and disability.

One of the most common areas of concern is lower back pain. It's a serious medical condition that's exacerbated by excess weight. Between 12 and 15 per cent of all annual healthcare visits are due to lower back pain. In the US alone, it's estimated the direct medical cost of lower back pain is US$85 billion. Take lost productivity into account and it's likely this cost increases to between $100 and $200 billion.

THE PLUSES OF GOOD POSTURE

If you spend extended periods of time sitting, it's easy to end up with postural problems; everything from hunching to stiff hips and knees.

One serious health issue related to bad posture is restricted breathing. When you're hunched forward, the movement of the ribcage is compromised making breathing shallow and frequent. This seriously affects your metabolic, cardiovascular and psychological health.

Another complication of rounded shoulders is neck pain, often caused by looking at a screen all day. To look straight ahead, we are forced to hyperextend our neck and contract the muscles of the cervical spine and shoulders. If this muscle contraction persists over time, chronic neck pain can result in muscle-tension headaches, nausea, dizziness, tingling in the hands and even chronic inflammation.

Bad posture also compromises your balance, which can lead to more falls and injuries, and can cause chronic pain in the back, neck, hips and knees. Posture also announces to the world who we are. Our presence – both physical and dynamic (the way we carry ourselves) – draws attention to us and influences those around us. Good bearing and posture echoes a good state of mind.

STRAIGHTEN UP

What is good posture? Your upper and lower body will be aligned with your centre of gravity, your neck is well centred on your shoulders, which should be relaxed and upright, your chest is open, the abdomen flat, and the pelvis, thighs and legs firmly on the ground below. Your weight should be distributed evenly across both feet, favouring neither the balls of the feet nor the heels. The same rules apply whether you are standing, walking or sitting.

A quick way to check whether your posture is good is to look at the soles of a pair of shoes you wear regularly. If they are more worn in the front, heels or the sides it means you could have an issue with your posture.

You should be able to comfortably stand with your back against a wall, legs slightly apart and rest your butt and shoulders against the wall so that the chest is open. Does your head touch the wall? If it doesn't, you could have a cervical vertebrae misalignment. Imagine a string pulling straight up from the top of your head and see if that allows your head to touch the wall. Now, breathe deeply into your diaphragm. That's correct posture.

Stretching before and after every exercise session assists with ease of movement and developing good posture. There's a range of simple stretches that can be incorporated into exercise routines, as well as at different points during the day when you've been sitting for prolonged periods.

There are other ways to straighten up, from taking yoga classes to joining exercise programs that deal specifically with posture.

HOW TO STRETCH

- You should never feel pain – only stretch to the limit at which you're comfortable.

- Slow down. Long, sustained stretches of at least 15 seconds, but preferably longer, are best for reducing muscle tightness.

- Breathe normally – never hold your breath while you're stretching.

- Stretching helps build back and neck muscle strength, which supports great posture.

- It also increases flexibility and movement of the joints.

- Stretching regularly will make you feel better.

STRETCH
HOLD EACH STRETCH FOR AT LEAST 15 SECONDS

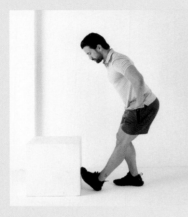

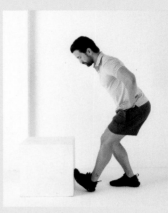

ANKLE/CALF STRETCH
Find a step or wall to place your foot against. Stretch for 15–20 seconds on each ankle. Repeat once with a straight front knee, once with a bent front knee.

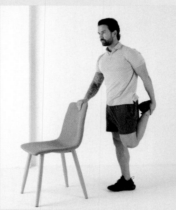

QUADRICEPS (FRONT OF THIGH) STRETCH
Aim to feel this in the front of the leg. Stand tall through the hips to deepen the stretch.

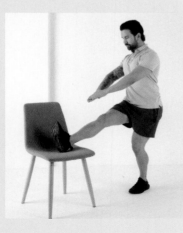

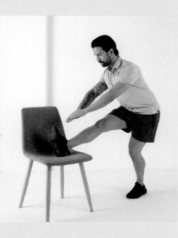

HAMSTRING STRETCH – STANDING, WITH A BENCH
Start with your foot resting on a chair or bench, toe pointing up and a slight bend in your knee (don't lock or overextend). Keep a straight back while leaning forward towards your toe.

HAMSTRING STRETCH – STANDING, NO BENCH

Start with your toe pointing up and a slight bend in your knee (don't lock or overextend). Keep a straight back while leaning forward towards your toe.

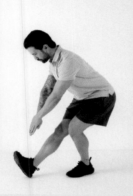

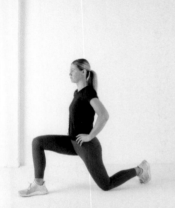

HIP FLEXOR STRETCH

Keeping your back straight and chest up, allow your hips to move forward until you feel a stretch at the front of the hip or thigh. You can intensify this stretch by raising your arm overhead on the same side as the back knee.

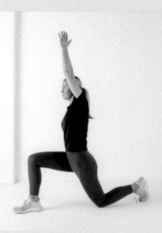

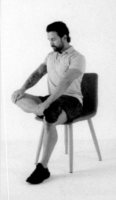

GLUTE STRETCH SEATED

Start with your ankle across the opposite knee, and hands stabilising both. Lean forward from the hips with a straight back to deepen the stretch.

STRETCH
HOLD EACH STRETCH FOR AT LEAST 15 SECONDS

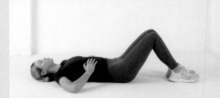 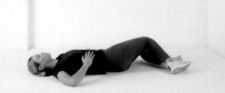

LOWER BACK STRETCH
Lying on your back, bend your knees to 90 degrees, feet slightly apart and on the ground. Let both knees fall across to one side until you feel a light stretch along the outside of your hip. Repeat on the other side.

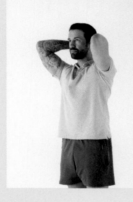 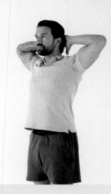

CHEST STRETCH
Keeping your neck firm and chest up, draw your elbows behind your head until you feel a stretch through the front of the shoulder and chest. Don't place pressure on your head and neck.

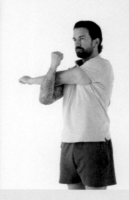

RHOMBOID (UPPER BACK) STRETCH
Aim to feel this stretch between your shoulder blades. Repeat on each side.

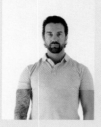 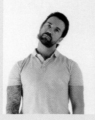 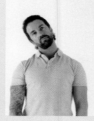

NECK STRETCH – EAR TO SHOULDER

Allow your ear to drop towards your shoulder until you feel a stretch.

NECK STRETCH – CHIN TO CHEST/LOOK UP

Keep shoulders back and chest up – don't round your back – look down and up.

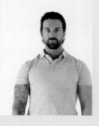 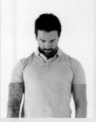 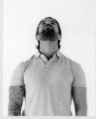

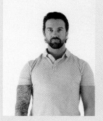 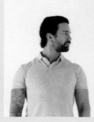

NECK STRETCH – LOOK OVER SHOULDER

Keep shoulders square, rotate head as far as you can comfortably until you feel the stretch.

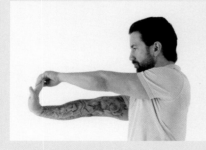 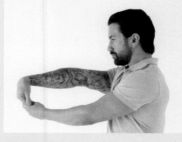

WRIST STRETCH – FLEX/EXTEND

With arm extended, gently draw your fingers of one hand back until you feel a stretch on the underside of your wrist. Repeat, folding your fingers below your wrist gently until you feel a stretch along the top of your wrist or forearm. Repeat on the other wrist.

EAST MEETS WEST

Say exercise and most people think of swimming laps at the pool, dawn runs and sessions at the gym. There is, however, a whole range of ancient Eastern disciplines that were designed to train both the mind and body.

Tai chi, for instance, which is based on the Taoist concept of yin and yang, is a form of harmonious movement, meditation and breathing. I like to think of it as a silent meditative dance. Practise it regularly and your body will become more agile and balanced, and you'll also feel a reduction in stress. Martial arts like taekwondo, aikido, judo and karate have similar benefits.

Probably the most commonly practised Eastern discipline, however, is yoga. There are many different styles of the ancient Indian doctrine that have been developed, but for improving overall health and bringing discipline and fortitude to the mind and body, I recommend Hatha yoga.

Hatha yoga consists of a series of exercises (called asanas) designed to train and balance every muscle of the body, and make both the body and mind stronger, more balanced and more resilient. Master expert B.K.S. Iyengar said it 'helped the lazy body to become active and vibrant'. Clinical studies have shown that practising Hatha yoga regularly for six months can reduce chronic back pain and improve flexibility and balance.

Find a good Hatha yoga teacher, practise the asanas regularly, and you'll see a rapid improvement in posture, flexibility, agility, coordination and mind-body harmony. It's the perfect exercise accompaniment for anyone, but especially people who have high-stress careers and spend a lot of time sitting at a desk.

Key to exercising is to make it a habit for life and you will feel the benefits every day.

YOGA

FOR POSTURE, BALANCE, FLEXIBILITY, AGILITY, COORDINATION AND MIND–BODY HARMONY

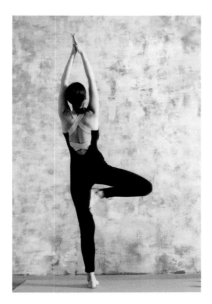

Vrikshasana or tree pose
Stand tall and straight with your arms at your sides. Bend your left knee and place your left foot high up on your thigh. The sole of your foot should be flat against your thigh. Once you are balanced, take a deep breath and raise your arms over your head from the side, and bring your palms together. Look straight ahead to keep your balance. While exhaling gently bring your hands back to your sides. Repeat with the right leg.

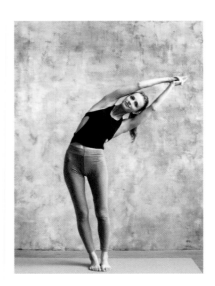

Parsva urdhva hastasana or upward salute side bend pose
Stand straight with feet together and arms beside you. Raise your arms over your head from the side, and bring your palms together above your head. Breathe in and imagine being pulled up by your hands. Bend leftwards from your waist. Hold for a few breaths and then return to standing. Repeat bending to the right side.

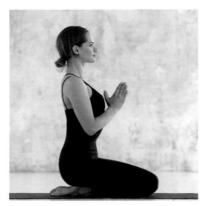

Vajrasana or thunderbolt pose

Kneel down and stretch the lower legs backwards while keeping them together. Gently lower your body so your thighs rest on the calf muscles. Raise your arms over your head from the side, and bring your palms together in front of your chest. Look straight ahead. Concentrate on your breathing. Hold for up to 5 minutes.

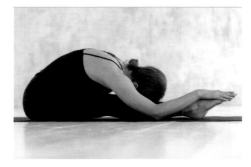

Paschimothanasana or seated forward bend

Lie flat on your back with legs close together. Slowly raise your head, chest and trunk until you are sitting up. Exhaling slowly, bend forward until you touch your toes. Hold this position for 10 seconds then slowly return to the upright position. Inhale. Lie back and relax.

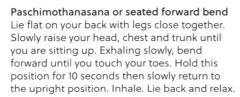

Vakrasana or half spinal twist

In a sitting position, bend your right leg and place the right heel near your left buttock. Place your left hand on the floor near your left thigh. Inhale and while exhaling twist your trunk and neck to the left, keeping the spine straight. Hold and breathe normally. Return to sitting by reversing the steps. Repeat from the opposite side.

Lotus pose

Sit on the floor with your legs straight out in front of you. Bend the left knee and hug it to your chest. Lean back slightly and bend the right leg and lift the left leg in front of the right. Hold and breathe normally.

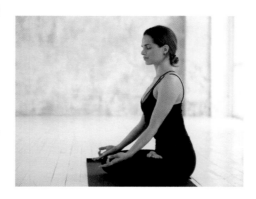

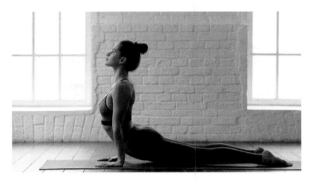

Bhujangasana or cobra pose

Lie on your stomach and place your forehead on the floor. Keep your feet hip-width apart and tops of your toes pressing the floor. Place your hands under your shoulders, keeping your elbows close to your body. Exhale as you lift your upper body, hold, then inhale as you lower your upper body to the floor.

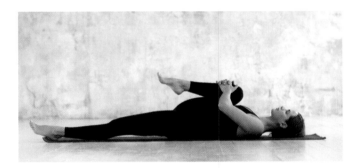

Apanasana or knees to chest pose

Lie on your back, stretching your legs out straight. Bend your right knee and draw it in towards your chest, holding it with your hands. Inhaling release the knee slightly away from your chest. Exhaling hug the knee to your chest. Repeat. Release your knee and return your leg to the floor. Repeat for the left knee, then repeat but draw both knees up to your chest.

Savangasana or supported shoulder stand pose

Lie on the floor, feet together and hands beside your body. Exhaling, slowly raise your legs up to perpendicular to the floor. Raise the lower portion of the trunk by pressing your hands under your hips and using your elbows as a fulcrum. Straighten your back. Your back is supported by your hands. Lift your trunk higher while your hands reach lower down your trunk towards your head. Your legs should be vertical. Hold for 5 minutes. Gently lower yourself by reversing the steps.

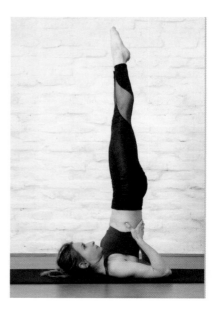

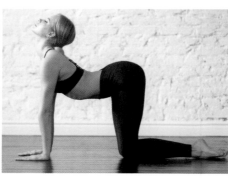

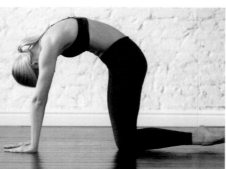

Bitilasana Marjaryasana or cat cow pose

Start on your hands and knees. As you inhale lift your buttocks upwards, your chest forward and allow you belly to sink. Lift your head, relax your shoulders away from your ears, and look straight ahead. As you exhale, start to arch your spine upward, tucking in your tail bone, and drawing your pubic bone forward. Release your head towards the floor and relax.

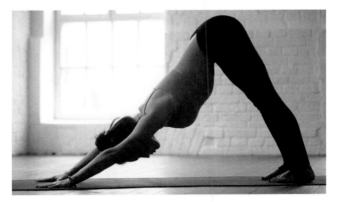

Adho Mukha Svanasana or downward-facing dog pose

Start on your hands and knees, with your hands slightly infront of your shoulders and knees below your hips. Turn your toes under and exhale as you lift your knees from the floor, stretching you heels toward the floor. Straighten your knees. Stay in the pose for 10 breaths, then bend your knees on exhalation and lower yourself down.

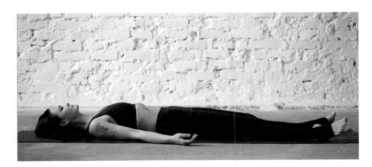

Savasana or corpse pose

Lie flat on your back while relaxing you body and mind. Close your eyes and focus on breathing naturally, and practise eliminating tension from your body.

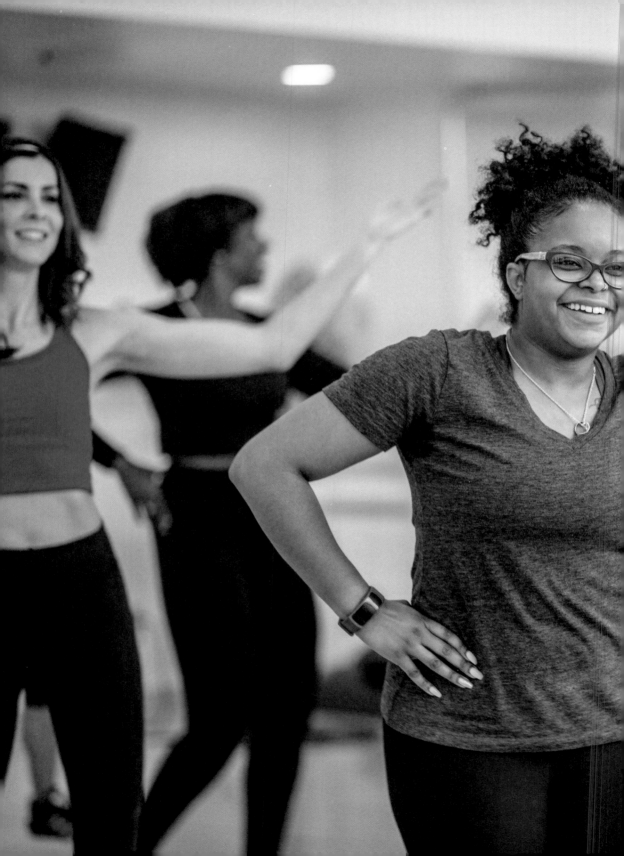

WEEKLY EXERCISE PROGRAM

DAY	AEROBIC	STRENGTH	FLEXIBILITY/ MOBILITY
DAY 1	30 minutes of your choice	30–45 minutes	5–10 minutes balance practice
DAY 2	30 minutes of your choice OR 20 minutes MIIT and 10 minutes warm up and cool down		5–10 minutes stretch
DAY 3	60 minutes low– medium intensity		5–10 minutes balance practice
DAY 4	30 minutes of your choice	30–45 minutes	5–10 minutes stretch
DAY 5	30 minutes of your choice OR 20 minute HIIT + 10 minute warm up and cool down		5–10 minutes balance practice
DAY 6	30–60 minute walk: moderate intensity	30–45 minutes (optional)	
DAY 7	30 minute walk		30 minutes stretch

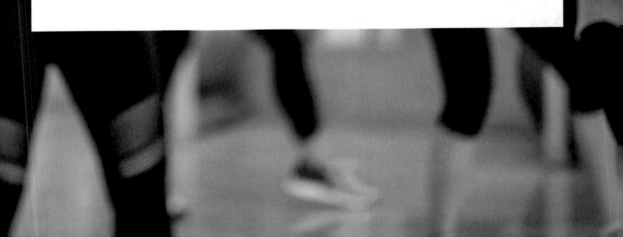

TAKE A BREATH

Slow, deep breathing is a powerful tool in fighting stress and anxiety. It's not that stress is always bad for us – it's a survival mechanism. If we're in danger, an automatic fight-or-flight response is triggered and our sympathetic nervous system kicks in: our heart rate swiftly speeds up and blood pressure spikes to deliver more blood and oxygen to the body so it can fight harder or flee faster.

That's great if you're being attacked by a dog, but if it's constantly prompted by money problems or family issues or a dissatisfying job, it's not. It can cause chronic and excessive activation of the sympathetic nervous system and cortisol systems leading to high blood pressure, immune suppression and cardiovascular disease. It can also promote accelerated ageing.

Deep breathing, typically performed during mindful meditation, tai chi or yoga, can stimulate the activity of the parasympathetic nervous system, which has the opposite effects of stress. Slow, deep breathing can significantly reduce blood pressure and mental stress, and augment heart rate variability and lower inflammation.

Start by practising for 5 to 10 minutes and progress to 15 minutes. Ideally perform your deep breathing at a set time every day. It's also helpful if you find yourself feeling particularly anxious at any point, such as before an exam or a job interview. It works like magic! It effectively 'tricks' your body and mind into believing it is relaxed. By calmly taking some long deep breaths, concentrating on the depth of the breaths, you will feel the calming and empowering effect it has.

WHEN STRESS IS BAD FOR YOU

Chronic stress and anxiety can result in irritability, muscle tension, headaches, poor concentration and sleepless nights. None of which makes for a happy and enjoyable life, but not only that, it can also cause serious chronic health problems and accelerate ageing.

THE RIGHT WAY TO BREATHE DEEPLY

Here's how to practise deep (diaphragmatic) breathing
and make it part of your day.

• Lie down on the floor, on your back, with your chest wide open and legs and arms slightly apart. Move around slightly until you feel comfortable and balanced. When you begin practising deep breathing, place your left hand on your abdomen so you can feel the movement of your diaphragm.

• Begin by simply observing your breath – the quality and symmetry of the inhalations and exhalations, and the sounds produced by the air entering and leaving your nostrils. After a couple of minutes your breath should become slower and slightly deeper.

• Now, take control. Let the air slowly fill the lowest part of your lungs so the abdomen moves out against your left hand.

• After a long, slow inhalation, with the abdomen fully dilated, exhale by engaging your abdominal muscles. Let them fall inward as you breathe slowly out your nose. At the end of the exhalation, gently spread your ribs ready for the next full inhalation.

• Keep taking deep breaths in and out, feeling your stomach rising and falling, smoothly and without interruptions. The movement of the abdomen and breath should be calm, natural and circular. If you begin to feel tension in your throat or temples, it indicates you're working too hard. Return to normal breathing until the tension subsides.

• At the conclusion of your deep-breathing session, return slowly and gently to the sitting position, keeping your eyes closed and your mind calm.

• Especially as this becomes more natural, you can add an 'aum' or 'om' to the final exhalations of your sessions. The vibrations of the sound will extend from your larynx to your brain. When you open your eyes again, it should feel as though you're waking from a deep sleep, with your mind clear and relaxed.

STEP THREE

WELLBEING

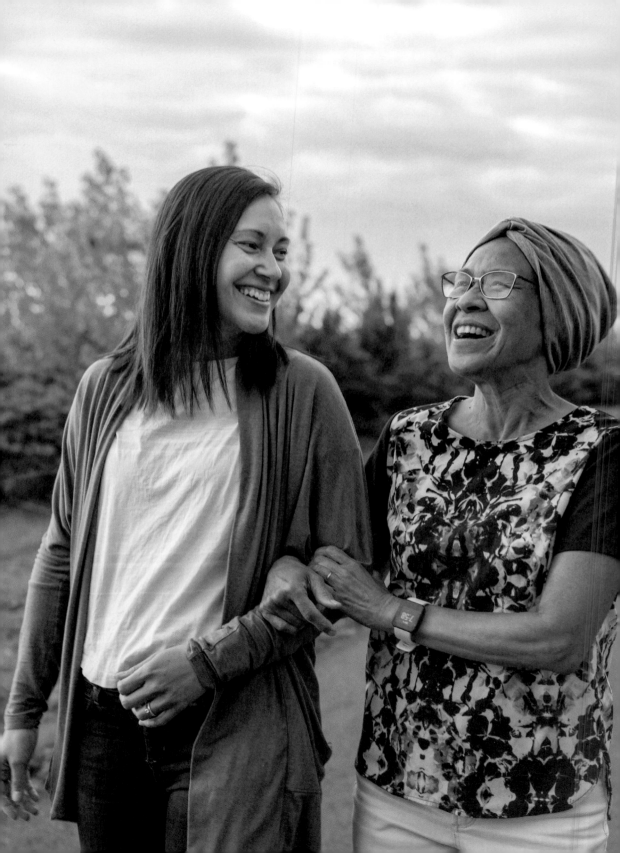

THINK YOUR WAY TO GOOD HEALTH: YOUR MIND AND SPIRITUAL HEALTH

While contemporary wellbeing tends to focus on the physical person and material needs, ancient medicine and philosophical systems always focused on the nourishment of the mind and soul. It's not enough to ensure you make a significant investment into nutrition and exercise. To create a healthy body that extends your chances of a long and disease-free life, you cannot ignore your mind because you will risk losing brain function and facing cognitive decline. Your emotional wellbeing and spiritual health are extremely important as well.

If you've already taken control of your nutrition choices and added good quality exercise to your routine, you'll already have started making improvements to your brain functioning and structure. Studies have shown that both a healthy diet and exercise are essential for preventing multiple strokes and dementia. There are, however, other important factors in preventing brain function disappearing – getting enough good quality sleep and reducing stress, maintaining connections with family, friends and the community and it's also important to keep adding to your brain bank.

It's not only about constantly learning and challenging your mind to ensure it doesn't lose its function. We also need to ensure that our social relationships, emotional health and spiritual and philosophical values are maintained – they play a significant role in staving off loneliness, depression and anger that can induce both metabolic and inflammatory alterations that lead to illness and an acceleration of the ageing process.

THE BRAIN THAT TRAINS

'The mind should not be idle, otherwise it will become
a dead tree and cold ash.'

Physician Cao Tingdong wrote those words hundreds of years ago in his text entitled *Maxims of Gerontology*. Then and now, doctors and scientists know that the brain – just like any bank account – needs to be fed regularly to ensure it doesn't decline with age. If you put a lot of money in the bank and just forget about it, fees will eat into the balance, and it will not grow and thrive. It's the same with your brain. We tend to do most of our learning in the first quarter or so of our lives, from the time we're toddlers until we finish university. Then a lot of us tend to coast along.

New cognitive stimuli and experiences cause a rearrangement of the connections between nerve cells and the architecture of our cerebral cortex. All that means is that – doing crosswords, playing board games, composing poetry, taking artistic photos, reading books, visiting museums and galleries, and attending interesting classes – makes us more able to keep the brain active and able to learn new skills.

Our brains have plasticity – it's especially prevalent in children, but fades with every passing year. The good news is that it can be improved, even in the elderly who are already showing early signs of dementia, and by exercising the mind you can improve cognitive function and memory. Some of the most effective methods for doing this tend to come from activities that use different parts of the brain, like learning a musical instrument or a foreign language.

There are also training programs, like sudoku, puzzles and computer games, that can improve memory and brain function. But it's also been shown that activities like yoga, tai chi, dance, playing chess and learning to draw, paint or sculpt can have a similar result.

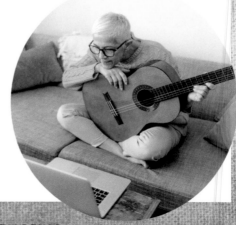

ALL ABOUT REST

While it's important to keep our minds active, it's equally important for brain health to ensure it gets good quality downtime. It is possible for our brains to become overstimulated, much the same way as it is possible to overtrain your body.

When we begin to suffer from mental fatigue – inability to concentrate, drowsiness, blurred vision – it's important to stop and rest. This can take the form of a short walk outside, a nap or a combination of both. Equally as important for those who tend to work in an office or at a desk is to improve how much you move and to add some vigorous exercise to your days. Perhaps that takes the form of housework or gardening on the weekend.

When it comes to brain regeneration, sleep is vitally important. Deep sleep is essential for memory, helping us to retain all the information we've learned during the day. During the day our conscious awareness can only concentrate on one thing at a time. When we sleep or meditate deeply, the brain acts more like a computer and is able to run multiple programs at once. The experiences we have during the day are consolidated in our long-term memory during deep sleep.

Even if there's no time for a nap, new studies show that short periods of wakeful rest – sitting quietly and relaxing – can help consolidate our memories, boost mental performance and improve our ability to master new information.

ARE YOU SLEEPING ENOUGH?

There is no magic number that works for everyone, but what is important is that you should be waking in the morning feeling recharged and invigorated. In general, however, adults should try to get between seven and eight hours of sleep each night.

Sleep deprivation is associated with a higher risk of obesity, diabetes, hypertension and cardiovascular disease. But it also has implications for our mental health, and can contribute to stress, depression, burnout and in the long run to dementia.

5 WAYS TO MORE HOURS AND DEEPER SLEEP EVERY NIGHT

1. **Blue light** The blue light emitted from LED screens and electronic devices disrupts the circadian rhythm of your brain and contributes to sleep disorders and insomnia. Turn devices off at least an hour before you go to bed.

2. **Exercise** Studies show that people who exercise regularly also spend increased hours in deep sleep. Exercise in the morning and you'll enhance your sleep that evening, but vigorous exercise in the evening can actually impair sleep quality.

3. **Meditation and yoga** There's growing evidence to suggest that doing Hatha yoga a couple of times a week and meditating, including deep breathing, can increase delta slow-wave sleep (the best kind).

4. **Learn something new** Mastering new tasks and learning new concepts — stimulating the brain and keeping it alert and active — during the day helps us to sleep at night.

5. **Listen to pink noise** Pink noise, which mimics the sounds of nature, can improve slow-wave deep sleep activity. There are apps that play different types of pink noise — ocean waves, a crackling fire, waterfalls, rain on the roof — that you can use as you're falling asleep.

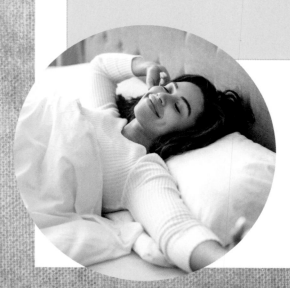

MINDFULNESS

There's so much going on in the world, competing for our attention, that it's easy to become distracted and unfocused. There's also often such a push towards success, many of us have numerous projects on the go and feel as though we have to schedule every minute of the day – building up anxiety. We forget to set aside time to relax and just be – to spend time in nature or enjoying the simple things in life.

Mindfulness may seem like a practice that's been developed to counteract the frenzied modern world, but in fact it is deeply rooted in the philosophy of Zen Buddhism. And it means to be conscious, focused and aware.

It's important for us, as participants in the modern world, to practice mindfulness daily. It turns off obsessive thinking, or what some call the monkey mind: a mind that rushes from one thought to another, worrying about the past and future. It's a type of anxiety that stops you from concentrating on what is happening right here, right now. You might also have found it means you can't get to sleep at night.

When you improve awareness by focusing on your thoughts, rather than getting carried away by them, it helps suppress negative emotions and stress. And it can help self-esteem and life satisfaction. Who doesn't want more of that?

PRACTICING THE ART OF NOW

Mindfulness exercises come in two parts.

The first is about focusing on the present moment, on what is happening to you and around you.

The second involves facing new experiences with curiosity and open-mindedness, without judgement, without trying to change their meaning or fighting against them. Even if it's something that may not seem pleasant, you need to approach it with a sense of inquisitiveness.

Practicing mindfulness is a way to become acquainted with observing what's going on around you without filtering your feelings or thoughts, or sorting them into what is good and what is bad. With time, you'll find you can just focus on the present moment, without lingering in the past or worrying about what will happen in the future. It'll allow you, when you feel distracted by your thoughts to refocus on your breathing, observe the breath, and return to the present.

BUT FIRST, SERENITY...

It's very possible that you may be reading this and considering mindfulness for the first time. While some progressive schools are now introducing meditation and mindfulness to the classroom, a lot of you might never have practiced either. But introducing regular mindfulness to your routine is important to create inner calm and peace of mind. It also helps us treat ourselves with kindness and enhances self-care and self-respect.

You are not your thoughts, and the sooner you are able to observe life from a wider perspective – almost as if you're stepping back from it and watching it from afar – the sooner you'll be able to improve the way you live your life. People who are able to do that can cope far better with stressful, sad or depressing experiences. They are able to be more resilient and not so easily discouraged.

There are plenty of benefits to embracing mindfulness – many of them already mentioned – but it can also help avoid unhealthy situations, such as overeating or drinking too much. Just as our bodies are more capable of fighting off infections and diseases when they are healthy, our minds, when they are calm and resilient, are better at fighting against adversity and negative experiences.

THE TEN BENEFITS OF MINDFULNESS

Incorporating meditation into your life every day has many benefits that extend well beyond each of your sessions.

1. Enhanced concentration.

Do you get easily distracted by whatever else is going on around you? Meditation will help you focus on what's important and to let go of internal and external distractions.

2. Decreased stress and anxiety.

Stress is the reaction to a perceived threat, and anxiety is a reaction to the stress itself. While regular aerobic exercise helps reduce both, mindful meditation has also been shown to decrease levels of tension, elevate and stabilise mood, and improve sleep. Additionally, deep breathing has been shown to powerfully reduce anxiety and stress.

3. Negative thoughts.

Constant negative thoughts about ourselves and our situation can result in consternation, fear and depression. Spend time ruminating over what's gone wrong in the past and you just end up unhappy. Mindfulness meditation is all about being in the present, and can help us focus on what's happening now rather than past or future events.

4. Reduced emotional reactivity.
How do you know when your mind is sound and healthy? Well, when you deal well with emotional challenges and 'bad' emotions like sadness, guilt, anger and fear. Studies have shown that regular meditation and mindfulness sessions can improve the stability of your emotions.

5. Increased flexible thinking.
This is just a fancy way of saying you adapt quickly to changes going on around you that you didn't anticipate. Say you're expecting a co-worker to have prepared a report for an important meeting you're presenting together. The day before, you find out they haven't finished it. Having good cognitive flexibility means you'll be able to disengage from the panic and find a solution. It lets you change gears without losing your cool.

6. Enhanced working memory.
Imagine your working memory as computer RAM – it allows your brain to store and manage new information while also learning, reasoning and working out what's going on around you. It only takes a short time once you've begun regular meditation training to improve memory and executive functioning.

7. Improved relationship satisfaction.
Do you feel as though you and your partner (or anyone else to whom you are close, for that matter) could communicate better? Perhaps you should practice mindfulness meditation together. It has an almost immediate short-term effect, improving relationship happiness and reducing stress, and in the longer term seems to enhance feelings of closeness and acceptance while cutting back conflict.

8. Increased empathy.
Because it stimulates the parts of our brain that control emotional processing, meditation can improve our compassion and warm-heartedness, and thus improve our ability to put ourselves in another's shoes.

9. Enhanced compassion for yourself. Not only does it help us empathise with others, but regular meditation helps us act more kindly towards ourselves. And people who have self-compassion have better relationships with others, more happiness and greater health.

10. Improved quality of life.
That's what you're here for, right? Mindful people have better intuition and self-insight, which in turn improves wellbeing and quality of life.

CALCULATING YOUR OWN MINDFULNESS

It's possibly not something you've really considered. You've probably never thought you needed to do it. But take the following assessment, called the Mindful, Attention and Awareness Scale (it was developed in 2003 by Professors Kirk W. Brown of the Virginia Commonwealth University and Richard M. Ryan of the University of Rochester), and give yourself a score from 1 (almost always) to 6 (almost never) for each statement.

1. I could be experiencing some emotion and not be conscious of it until sometime later.
2. I break or spill things because of carelessness, not paying attention, or thinking of something else.
3. I find it difficult to stay focused on what's happening in the present.
4. I tend to walk quickly to get where I'm going without paying attention to what I experience along the way.
5. I tend not to notice feelings of physical tension or discomfort until they really grab my attention.
6. I forget a person's name almost as soon as I've been told it for the first time.
7. It seems as if I am 'running on automatic' without much awareness of what I'm doing.
8. I rush through activities without being really attentive to them.
9. I get so focused on the goal I want to achieve that I lose touch with what I am doing right now to get there.
10. I do jobs or tasks automatically, without being aware of what I'm doing.
11. I find myself listening to someone with one ear, doing something else at the same time.
12. I drive places on 'automatic pilot' and then wonder why I went there.
13. I find myself preoccupied with the future or the past.
14. I find myself doing things without paying attention.
15. I snack without being aware that I am eating.

How did you go? Add up your scores then get an average by dividing by 15. A high score indicates attentiveness and a more present awareness, while a low score indicates you're not really mindful of what's happening in the present. Everyone can benefit from regular mindfulness practice, but in particular it's important for those who tend to live their life on automatic.

GETTING INTO MINDFULNESS

You don't have to spend months in an ashram in India to begin a life-altering meditation practice. You can practice mindfulness anywhere and at any time. If you walk part of the way to work or spend some of your day each week doing the housework, you can even utilise that time.

When you're getting started, it's great to find a nice quiet place with no distractions, and to set aside the same time each day so that you get into a routine. It might be before you start your day or after you've had a shower in the evening.

Sit on a comfortable chair or lie down on the bed. For a full three minutes, observe your breathing. Focus your full attention on the air entering your nose, your ribcage expanding and contracting, the air flowing in and out of your body. Just be a spectator. Don't make any judgements. Don't change the rhythm of your breathing. Just observe.

If your mind begins to wander, gently try to bring your thoughts back to your breathing. Once you get better at this, you can use it at any time – even while you're sitting at your desk at work – you start to feel a little stressed or anxious.

TAKE IT OUTSIDE

Another lovely mindfulness exercise can be done whenever you're outside. If you're in the park, watch a bird, listen to leaves fluttering or observe a cloud moving across the sky. Watch it carefully for two or three minutes, without doing anything. Relax and try to bring your mind into harmony with whatever it is you're observing.

If it starts to wander – you begin thinking about a project at work, an argument you had with your mother, or what you're having for dinner – bring your attention back to the bird or cloud and start over.

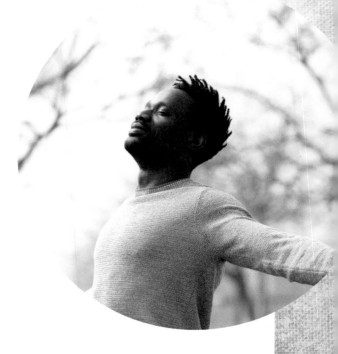

FEEL THE SENSATION

A third easy mindfulness exercise is to focus on the sensations when you drink or eat something delicious, like a piece of fruit. For instance, if you're going to eat a strawberry, think about where it was grown, its colour and its shape. Run your fingers over it and feel its texture, notice its aroma. How does it feel on your lips? How does it taste on your tongue? Eat it slowly and experience all its flavours. You can do the same when you're sipping green tea.

These really simple exercises can make you aware of just how often you would normally do these things on autopilot, without any connection to the experience. Reconnecting to everything around you helps you to live in the moment and take nothing for granted.

At the end of each mindfulness exercise, take three to five minutes to do some deep diaphragmatic breathing (as explained on page 197). This will have a calming effect that can either help you get on with your day or sleep more soundly. Which is also why you should take a few slow, deep breaths whenever you are feeling stressed.

POSITIVE RELATIONSHIPS

Positive relationships with family and friends play an important role in promoting health, both physical and emotional. You need a sense of belonging to feel good – social isolation or a lack of ties can be painful for many people. Those of us who have a rich network of friends and family, who trust and support each other, have lower levels of depression and anxiety and are healthier than those who are selfish or socially isolated. We're also more likely to have empathy for both others and ourselves.

HELPING HAPPINESS FLOURISH

Happiness means different things to different people. Lots of people associate money with happiness, but while you might get a flash of joy from buying a new car or a beautiful dress, it is sure to be fleeting.

It would be difficult to be happy or content if we were unwell, in pain or having emotional difficulties. Taking positive steps towards ensuring both your body and mind are healthy – through good nutrition, regular exercise, mindfulness and a positive spiritual and philosophical stance – will have a direct effect on your happiness levels. But there are other ways to inflate your levels of wellbeing.

Get back to nature Whenever you can, spend time in the great outdoors. Walking in a park, hiking in the mountains or swimming in the ocean will remind you of the unlimited reserve of universal energy. Admire your surroundings and breathe in the fresh air.

Immerse yourself in creativity It's great to devote time to artistic and creative disciplines, whether you take up painting, write poetry or join a local amateur theatre group. Even turning on a favourite song and singing and dancing to it can give you a boost.

Channel compassion Serenity is destroyed by anger, fear and egoism, but if you develop your ability to feel at peace with yourself and develop altruism and compassion for others you'll become empowered. It's important to do so to enhance happiness.

Opt for optimism Whenever you can, smile. Looking on the bright side helps your mood and your smile helps inject positivity into interactions you have with those around you. Start to ponder the deeper aspects of your life by reading about philosophy or spirituality, and take part in contemplative activities, like yoga and meditation. The positive vibrations you'll begin to emanate will help both you and everyone around you.

Discover your purpose When your life means something and you're working on projects that have a purpose, you'll undoubtedly feel more fulfilled. It's important to create or contribute to something that is about more than your own ego and add to society in some way. Useful and altruistic activities promote positive emotions and profound social connections, both of which help us feel satisfied with our lives.

ONE STEP AT A TIME

All of this probably seems like a lot. Changing what you eat, adding exercise to our life, becoming more mindful, seeking out ways to make ourselves happier... It might even seem like such a huge investment that it's enough to scare you off.

Don't despair. You will need some patience and determination, but making small, incremental contributions towards your ongoing health will lead to an almost immediate improvement to your wellbeing.

The path to health, self-awareness and spiritual richness is a long one, and you'll need to keep following it for the rest of your life. But make a start now and you'll reduce the risk of becoming sick and move towards living a long, creative and fulfilling life with your friends and loved ones.

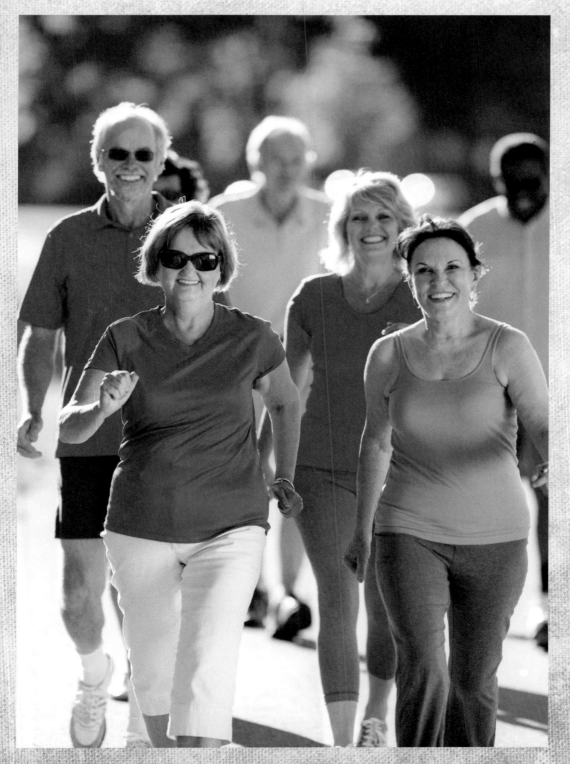

ACKNOWLEDGEMENTS

This book would not be possible without the love and support of my beloved mother Antonietta Iozzi, my dear son Lorenzo and my wife Laura Piccio.

There are many others who have inspired and supported me in this amazing journey of discovery. A special thanks to my uncle Francesco who introduced me to many enlightening philosophical and traditional medicine books, including the *Tao Te Ching*, the *Chuang Tzu*, the *I Ching*, the *Upanishads*, the *Yellow Emperor's Classic of Medicine* and the *Yoga Sutra of Patañjali*. He also led me to more modern interpretations, such as the *Manual of Zen Buddhism* by DT Suzuki, *Total Freedom* by Jiddu Krishnamurti, and the *Art of Yoga* by B.K.S. Iyengar.

Critical support came from my mentors and dear friends Professors John O. Holloszy, Giampaolo Velo, Franco Salvatore and Sergio Pecorelli.

I have also to thank the many postdoctoral fellows, PhD students and medical students who were critical to my lab's success. In particular, I would like to thank and acknowledge the help of Andrew Greig, a personal trainer and medical student, who helped me write the exercise program section of this book.

A special thank you goes to my publisher, Pam Brewster, who worked closely with me for almost a year crafting this more practical book that complements my previous theoretical one, *The Path to Longevity*.

LUIGI FONTANA

Professor Luigi Fontana is the world's foremost authority in human healthy longevity. His pioneering studies on the effects of dietary restriction, fasting, diet composition and exercise training have opened new areas of research that holds incredible promise for the prevention of age-related chronic illnesses and for the elucidation of the mechanisms that can slow human ageing.

Professor Fontana has worked in some of the world's finest medical institutions, including two that have produced multiple Nobel Laureate, Washington University in St Louis (USA) and the Italian Institute of Health in Rome, Italy.

In 2018, Professor Fontana was recruited to the University of Sydney as the Leonard P. Ullmann Chair of Translational Metabolic Health and Director of the Healthy Longevity Research and Clinical Program. He is also the Scientific Director of the Charles Perkins Centre Royal Prince Alfred Clinic, and a clinical academic in the Department of Endocrinology at Royal Prince Alfred Hospital in Sydney, where he continues his clinical practice and research into health, wellbeing and disease prevention.

His work has been published in more than 140 highly cited academic papers in prestigious journals, including *Science*, *Nature*, *Cell* and *New England Journal of Medicine* among many others. Professor Fontana has also presented his work at more than 250 international conferences and top medical schools and research institutes around the world.

Professor Fontana believes that, as a society, we urgently need to transition from a primarily disease-centered medical system to a balanced preventative and personalised treatment healthcare system. This involves people making choices that will set themselves up for long, healthy and happy lives, while contributing to the protection of the environment. Those already suffering from chronic conditions, including obesity, hypertension, diabetes, heart disease, cancer, autoimmune and allergic disorders, and emotional and psychological distress, can also make positive changes that will have a beneficial influence on their lives.

This is the work covered in this book, with Professor Fontana sharing practical information that has proven invaluable to him, his family and friends, and to the patients he's treated. These are the steps you can incorporate into your life to avoid a wide range of physical and emotional afflictions and create a longer and healthier life for yourself.

Published in 2023 by Hardie Grant Books,
an imprint of Hardie Grant Publishing

Hardie Grant Books (Melbourne)
Wurundjeri Country
Building 1, 658 Church Street
Richmond, Victoria 3121

Hardie Grant Books (London)
5th & 6th Floors
52–54 Southwark Street
London SE1 1UN

hardiegrant.com/au/books

Hardie Grant acknowledges the Traditional Owners of the country on which we work, the Wurundjeri
people of the Kulin nation and the Gadigal people of the Eora nation, and recognises their continuing
connection to the land, waters and culture. We pay our respects to their Elders past and present.

A catalogue record for this
book is available from the
NATIONAL LIBRARY OF AUSTRALIA National Library of Australia

Manual of Healthy Longevity & Wellbeing
ISBN 9781743796825

10 9 8 7 6 5 4 3 2 1

Publisher: Pam Brewster
Cover designer: Luke Causby, Blue Cork
Text designer: Hannah Schubert
Recipe photographer: Bonnie Savage
Recipe stylist: Leesa O'Reilly
Additional images: istock, Getty images
Exercise photographer: Bonnie Savage
Exercise supervision and advice: Andrew Grieg, BSc(Adv) MExSc MBiotechMComm
Exercise photoshoot: Joey Philpot, Elise Embrey. Thanks to AUSactive and Billie Cox.
Design manager: Kristin Thomas
Production manager: Todd Rechner

Colour reproduction by Splitting Image Colour Studio
Printed in China by Leo Paper Products LTD.